VET IN A SPIN

James Herriot grew up in Glasgow and qualified as a veterinary surgeon at Glasgow Veterinary College. Shortly afterwards, he took up a position as an assistant in a North Yorkshire practice where he remained, with the exception of his wartime service in the RAF, until his death in 1995.

JAMES HERRIOT

VET IN A SPIN

PAN BOOKS

First published 1977 by Michael Joseph Ltd

First published in paperback 1978 by Pan Books

This edition published 2006 by Pan Books
an imprint of Pan Macmillan Ltd
Pan Macmillan, 20 New Wharf Road, London N1 9RR
Basingstoke and Oxford
Associated companies throughout the world
www.panmacmillan.com

ISBN 978-0-330-44357-9

3 5 7 9 8 6 4

A CIP catalogue record for this book is available from
the British Library.

Printed and bound in Great Britain by
Mackays of Chatham plc, Chatham, Kent

Visit **www.panmacmillan.com** to read more about all our books and to buy
them. You will also find features, author interviews and news of any author
events, and you can sign up for e-newsletters so that you're always first to hear
about our new releases.

With love to

ROSIE, JIM and GILL

1

This was a very different uniform. The wellingtons and breeches of my country vet days seemed far away as I climbed into the baggy flying suit and pulled on the sheepskin boots and the gloves – the silk ones first then the big clumsy pair on top. It was all new but I had a feeling of pride.

Leather helmet and goggles next, then I fastened on my parachute, passing the straps over my shoulders and between my legs and buckling them against my chest before shuffling out of the flight hut on to the long stretch of sunlit grass.

Flying Officer Woodham was waiting for me there. He was to be my instructor and he glanced at me apprehensively as though he didn't relish the prospect. With his dark boyish good looks he resembled all the pictures I had seen of Battle of Britain pilots and in fact, like all our instructors, he had been through this crisis in our history. They had been sent here as a kind of holiday after their tremendous experience but it was said that they regarded their operations against the enemy as a picnic compared with this. They had faced the might of the Luftwaffe without flinching but we terrified them.

As we walked over the grass I could see one of my friends coming in to land. The little biplane slewed and weaved crazily in the sky. It just missed a clump of trees, then about fifty feet from the ground it dropped like a stone, bounced high on its wheels, bounced twice again then zig-zagged to a halt. The helmeted head in the rear cockpit jerked and nodded as though it were making some pointed remarks to the head in front. Flying Officer Woodham's face was expressionless but I knew what he was thinking. It was his turn next.

The Tiger Moth looked very small and alone on the wide stretch of green. I climbed up and strapped myself into the cockpit while my instructor got in behind me. He went through the drill which I would soon know by heart like a piece of poetry. A fitter gave the propeller a few turns for priming. Then 'Contact!', the fitter swung the prop, the engine roared, the chocks were pulled away from the wheels and we were away, bumping over the grass, then suddenly and miraculously lifting and soaring high over the straggle of huts into the summer sky with the patchwork of the soft countryside of southern England unfolding beneath us.

I felt a sudden elation, not just because I liked the sensation but because I had waited so long for this moment. The months of drilling and marching and studying navigation had been leading up to the time when I would take to the air and now it had arrived.

FO Woodham's voice came over the intercom. 'Now you've got her. Take the stick and hold her steady. Watch the artificial horizon and keep it level. See that cloud ahead? Line yourself up with it and keep your nose on it.'

I gripped the joystick in my gauntleted hand. This was lovely. And easy, too. They had told me flying would be a simple matter and they had been right. It was child's play. Cruising along I glanced down at the grandstand of Ascot racecourse far below.

I was just beginning to smile happily when a voice crashed in my ear. 'Relax, for God's sake! What the hell are you playing at?'

I couldn't understand him. I felt perfectly relaxed and I thought I was doing fine, but in the mirror I could see my instructor's eyes glaring through his goggles.

'No, no, no! That's no bloody good! Relax, can't you hear me, relax!'

'Yes, sir,' I quavered and immediately began to stiffen up. I couldn't imagine what was troubling the man but as I began to stare with increasing desperation, now at the artificial horizon, then at the nose of the aircraft against the cloud ahead, the noises over the intercom became increasingly apoplectic.

I didn't seem to have a single problem, yet all I could hear were curses and groans and on one occasion the voice rose to a scream. 'Get your bloody finger out, will you!'

I stopped enjoying myself and a faint misery welled in me. And as always when that happened I began to think of Helen and the happier life I had left behind. In the open cockpit the wind thundered in my ears, lending vivid life to the picture forming in my mind.

The wind was thundering here, too, but it was against the window of our bedsitter. It was early November and a golden autumn had changed with brutal suddenness to arctic cold. For two weeks an icy rain had swept the grey towns and villages which huddled in the folds of the Yorkshire Dales, turning the fields into shallow lakes and the farmyards into squelching mud-holes.

Everybody had colds. Some said it was flu, but whatever it was it decimated the population. Half of Darrowby seemed to be in bed and the other half sneezing at each other.

I myself was on a knife edge, crouching over the fire, sucking an antiseptic lozenge and wincing every time I had to swallow. My throat felt raw and there was an ominous tickling at the back of my nose. I shivered as the rain hurled a drumming cascade of water against the glass. I was all alone in the practice. Siegfried had gone away for a few days and I just daren't catch cold.

It all depended on tonight. If only I could stay indoors and then have a good sleep I could throw this off, but as I glanced over at the phone on the bedside table it looked like a crouching beast ready to spring.

Helen was sitting on the other side of the fire, knitting. She didn't have a cold – she never did. And even in those early days of our marriage I couldn't help feeling it was a little unfair. Even now, thirty-five years later, things are just the same and, as I go around sniffling, I still feel tight-lipped at her obstinate refusal to join me.

I pulled my chair closer to the blaze. There was always a lot of night work in our kind of practice but maybe I would be lucky. It was eight o'clock with never a cheep, and perhaps fate had decreed that I would not be hauled out into that sodden darkness in my weakened state.

Helen came to the end of a row and held up her knitting. It was a sweater for me, about half done.

'How does it look, Jim?' she asked.

I smiled. There was something in her gesture that seemed to epitomize our life together. I opened my mouth to tell her it was simply smashing when the phone pealed with a suddenness which made me bite my tongue.

Tremblingly I lifted the receiver while horrid visions of calving heifers floated before me. An hour with my shirt off would just tip me nicely over the brink.

'This is Sowden of Long Pasture,' a voice croaked.

'Yes, Mr Sowden ?' I gripped the phone tightly. I would know my fate in a moment.

'I 'ave a big calf 'ere. Looks very dowly and gruntin' bad. Will ye come ?'

A long breath of relief escaped me. A calf with probable stomach trouble. It could have been a lot worse.

'Right, I'll see you in twenty minutes,' I said.

As I turned back to the cosy warmth of the little room the injustice of life smote me.

'I've got to go out, Helen.'

'Oh, no.'

'Yes, and I have this cold coming on,' I whimpered. 'And just listen to that rain.'

'Yes, you must wrap up well, Jim.'

I scowled at her. 'That place is ten miles away, and a cheerless dump if ever there was one. There's not a warm corner anywhere.' I fingered my aching throat. 'A trip out there's just what I need – I'm sure I've got a temperature.' I don't know if all veterinary surgeons blame their wives when they get an unwanted call, but heaven help me, I've done it all my life.

Instead of giving me a swift kick in the pants Helen smiled up at me. 'I'm really sorry, Jim, but maybe it won't take you long. And you can have a bowl of hot soup when you get back.'

I nodded sulkily. Yes, that was something to look forward to. Helen had made some brisket broth that day, rich and meaty, crowded with celery. leeks and carrots and with a flavour to bring a man back from the dead. I kissed her and trailed off into the night.

Long Pasture Farm was in the little hamlet of Dowsett and I had travelled this narrow road many times. It snaked its way high into the wild country and on summer days the bare lonely hills had a serene beauty; treeless and austere, but with a clean wind sweeping over the grassy miles.

But tonight as I peered unhappily through the streaming wind-screen the unseen surrounding black bulk pressed close and I could imagine the dripping stone walls climbing high to the summits where the rain drove across the moorland, drenching the heather and bracken, churning the dark mirrors of the bog water into liquid mud.

When I saw Mr Sowden I realized that I was really quite fit. He had obviously been suffering from the prevalent malady for some time, but like most farmers he just had to keep going at his hard ceaseless work. He looked at me from swimming eyes, gave a couple of racking coughs that almost tore him apart and led me into the buildings. He held an oil lamp high as we entered a lofty barn and in the feeble light I discerned various rusting farm implements, a heap of potatoes and another of turnips and in a corner a makeshift pen where my patient stood.

It wasn't the two-week-old baby calf I had half expected, but a little animal of six months, almost stirk age, but not well grown. It had all the signs of a 'bad doer' – thin and pot-bellied with its light roan coat hanging in a thick overgrown fringe below its abdomen.

'Allus been a poor calf,' Mr Sowden wheezed between coughs. 'Never seemed to put on flesh. Rain stopped for a bit this afternoon, so ah let 'im out for a bit of fresh air and now look at 'im.'

I climbed into the pen and as I slipped the thermometer into the rectum I studied the little creature. He offered no resistance as I gently pushed him to one side, his head hung down and he gazed apathetically at the floor from deep sunk eyes. Worst of all was the noise he was making. It was more than a grunt – rather a long, painful groan repeated every few seconds.

'It certainly looks like his stomach,' I said. 'Which field was he in this afternoon?'

'I nobbut let 'im have a walk round t'orchard for a couple of hours.'

'I see.' I looked at the thermometer. The temperature was subnormal. 'I suppose there's a bit of fruit lying around there.'

Mr Sowden went into another paroxysm, then leaned on the boards of the pen to recover his breath. 'Aye, there's apples and pears all over t'grass. Had a helluva crop this year.'

I put the stethoscope over the rumen and instead of the normal surge and bubble of the healthy stomach I heard only a deathly silence. I palpated the flank and felt the typical doughy fullness of impaction.

'Well, Mr Sowden, I think he's got a bellyful of fruit and it's brought his digestion to a complete halt. He's in a bad way.'

The farmer shrugged. 'Well, if 'e's just a bit bunged up, a good dose of linseed oil 'ud shift 'im.'

'I'm afraid it's not as simple as that,' I said. 'This is a serious condition.'

'Well, what are we goin' to do about it, then?' He wiped his nose and looked at me morosely.

I hesitated. It was bitterly cold in the old building and already I was feeling shivery and my throat ached. The thought of Helen and the bedsitter and the warm fire was unbearably attractive. But I had seen impactions like this before and tried treating them with purgatives and it didn't work. This animal's temperature was falling to the moribund level and he had a sunken eye – if I didn't do something drastic he would be dead by morning.

'There's only one thing will save him,' I said. 'And that's a rumenotomy.'

'A what?'

'An operation. Open up his first stomach and clear out all the stuff that shouldn't be there.'

'Are you sure? D'ye not think a good pint of oil would put 'im right. It 'ud be a lot easier.'

It would indeed. For a moment the fireside and Helen glowed like a jewel in a cave, then I glanced at the calf. Scraggy and long-haired, he looked utterly unimportant, infinitely vulnerable and dependent. It would be the easiest thing in the world to leave him groaning in the dark till morning.

'I'm quite sure, Mr Sowden. He's so weak that I think I'll do it under a local anaesthetic, so we'll need some help.'

The farmer nodded slowly. 'Awright, ah'll go down t'village and get George Hindley.' He coughed again, painfully. 'But by gaw, ah could do without this tonight. Ah'm sure I've got brown chitis.'

Brown chitis was a common malady among the farmers of those days and there was no doubt this poor man was suffering from it but my pang of sympathy faded as he left because he took the lamp with him and the darkness closed tightly on me.

There are all kinds of barns. Some of them are small, cosy and fragrant with hay, but this was a terrible place. I had been in here on sunny afternoons and even then the dank gloom of crumbling walls and rotting beams was like a clammy blanket and all warmth and softness seemed to disappear among the cobwebbed rafters high above. I used to feel that people with starry-eyed notions of farming ought to take a look inside that barn. It was evocative of the grim comfortless other side of the agricultural life.

I had it to myself now, and as I stood there listening to the wind rattling the door on its latch a variety of draughts whistled round me and a remorseless drip-drip from the broken pantiles on the roof sent icy droplets trickling over my head and neck. And as the minutes ticked away I began to hop from foot to foot in a vain effort to keep warm.

Dales farmers are never in a hurry and I hadn't expected a quick return, but after fifteen minutes in the impenetrable blackness bitter thoughts began to assail me. Where the hell was the man? Maybe he and George Hindley were brewing a pot of tea for themselves or perhaps settling down to a quick game of dominoes. My legs were trembling by the time the oil lamp reappeared in the entrance and Mr Sowden ushered his neighbour inside.

'Good evening, George,' I said. 'How are you?'

'Only moderate, Mr Herriot,' the newcomer sniffled. 'This bloody caud's just – ah – ah – whooosh – just getting' a haud o' me.' He blew lustily into a red handkerchief and gazed at me blearily.

I looked around me. 'Well let's get started. We'll need an operating table. Perhaps you could stack up a few straw bales?'

The two men trailed out and returned, carrying a couple of bales apiece. When they were built up they were about the right height but rather wobbly.

'We could do with a board on top.' I blew on my freezing fingers and stamped my feet. 'Any ideas?'

Mr Sowden rubbed his chin. 'Aye, we'll get a door.' He shuffled out into the yard with his lamp and I watched him struggling to lift one of the cow byre doors from its hinges. George went to give him a hand and as the two of them pulled and heaved I thought wearily that veterinary operations didn't trouble me all that much but getting ready for them was a killer.

Finally the men staggered back into the barn, laid the door on top of the bales and the theatre was ready.

'Let's get him up,' I gasped.

We lifted the unresisting little creature on to the improvised table and stretched him on his right side. Mr Sowden held his head while George took charge of the tail and the rear end.

Quickly I laid out my instruments, removed coat and jacket and rolled up my shirt sleeves. 'Damn! We've no hot water. Will you bring some, Mr Sowden?'

I held the head and again waited interminably while the farmer went to the house. This time it was worse without my warm clothing, and cold ate into me as I pictured the farm kitchen and the slow scooping of the water from the side boiler into a bucket, then the unhurried journey back to the buildings.

When Mr Sowden finally reappeared I added antiseptic to the bucket and scrubbed my arms feverishly. Then I clipped the hair on the left side and filled the syringe with local anaesthetic. But as I infiltrated the area I felt my hopes sinking.

'I can hardly see a damn thing.' I looked helplessly at the oil lamp balanced on a nearby turnip chopper. 'That light's in the wrong place.'

Wordlessly Mr Sowden left his place and began to tie a length of plough cord to a beam. He threw it over another beam and made it fast before suspending the lamp above the calf. It was a big improvement but it took a long time, and by the time he had finished I had abandoned all hope of ever throwing off my cold. I was frozen right through and a burning sensation had started in my chest. I would soon be in the same state as my helpers. Brown chitis was just round the corner.

Anyway, at least I could start now, and I incised skin, muscles, peritoneum and rumenal wall at record speed. I plunged an arm deep into the opened organ, through the fermenting mass of stomach contents, and in a flash all my troubles dissolved. Along the floor of the rumen apples and pears were spread in layers, some of them bitten but most of them whole and intact. Bovines take most of their food in big swallows and chew it over later at their leisure, but no animal could make cud out of this lot.

I looked up happily. 'It's just as I thought. He's full of fruit.'

'Hhrraaagh!' replied Mr Sowden. Coughs come in various forms but this one was tremendous and fundamental, starting at the soles of his hob-nailed boots and exploding right in my face.

I hadn't realized how vulnerable I was with the farmer leaning over the calf's neck, his head a few inches from mine. 'Hhrraaagh!' he repeated, and a second shower of virus-laden moisture struck me. Apparently Mr Sowden either didn't know or didn't care about droplet infection, but with my hands inside my patient there was nothing I could do about it.

Instinctively I turned my face a little in the other direction.

'Whoosh!' went George. It was a sneeze rather than a cough, but it sent a similar deadly spray against my other cheek. I realized there was no escape. I was hopelessly trapped between the two of them.

But as I say, my morale had received a boost. Eagerly I scooped out great handfuls of the offending fruit and within minutes the floor of the barn was littered with Bramley's seedlings and Conference pears.

'Enough here to start a shop,' I laughed.

'Hhrraaagh!' responded Mr Sowden.

'Whooosh!' added George, not to be outdone.

When I had sent the last apple and pear rolling into the darkness I scrubbed up again and started to stitch. This is the longest and most wearisome part of a rumenotomy. The excitement of diagnosis and discovery is over and it is a good time for idle chat, funny stories, anything to pass the time.

But there in the circle of yellow light with the wind whirling round my feet from the surrounding gloom and occasional icy trickles of rain running down my back I was singularly short of gossip, and my companions, sunk in their respective miseries, were in no mood for badinage.

I was halfway down the skin sutures when a tickle mounted at the back of my nose and I had to stop and stand upright.

'Ah – ah – ashooo!' I rubbed my forearm along my nose.

'He's startin',' murmured George with mournful satisfaction.

'Aye, 'e's off,' agreed Mr Sowden, brightening visibly.

I was not greatly worried. I had long since come to the conclusion that my cause was lost. The long session of freezing in my shirt sleeves would have done it without the incessant germ bombardment from either side. I was resigned to my fate and besides, when I inserted the last stitch and helped the calf down from that table I felt a deep thrill of satisfaction. That horrible groan had vanished and the little animal was looking around him as though he had been away for a while. He wasn't cheerful yet, but I knew his pain had gone and that he would live.

'Bed him up well, Mr Sowden.' I started to wash my instruments in the bucket. 'And put a couple of sacks round him to keep him warm. I'll call in a fortnight to take out the stitches.'

The fortnight seemed to last a long time. My cold, as I had confidently expected, developed into a raging holocaust which settled down into the inevitable brown chitis with an accompanying cough which rivalled Mr Sowden's.

Mr Sowden was never an ebullient man but I expected him to look a little happier when I removed the stitches. Because the calf was bright and lively I had to chase him around his pen to catch him.

Despite the fire in my chest I had that airy feeling of success.

'Well,' I said expansively. 'He's done very well. He'll make a good bullock some day.'

The farmer shrugged gloomily. 'Aye, reckon 'e will. But there was no need for all that carry on.'

'No need . . . ?'

'Naw. Ah've been talkin' to one or two folk about t'job and they all said it was daft to open 'im up like that. Ah should just 'ave given 'im a pint of oil like I said.'

'Mr Sowden, I assure you . . .'

'And now ah'll have a big bill to pay.' He dug his hands deep into his pockets.

'Believe me, it was worth it.'

'Nay, nay, never.' He started to walk away, then looked over his shoulder. 'It would've been better if you 'adn't come.'

I had done three circuits with FO Woodham and on this third one he had kept fairly quiet. Obviously I was doing all right now and I could start enjoying myself again. Flying was lovely.

The voice came over the intercom again. 'I'm going to let you land her yourself this time. I've told you how to do it. Right, you've got her.'

'I've got her,' I replied. He had indeed told me how to do it – again and again – and I was sure I would have no trouble.

As we lost height the tops of the trees appeared, then the

grass of the airfield came up to meet us. It was the moment of truth. Carefully I eased the stick back, then at what I thought was the right moment I slammed it back against my stomach. Maybe a bit soon because we bounced a couple of times and that made me forget to seesaw the rudder bar so that we careered from side to side over the turf before coming to a halt.

With the engine stilled I took a deep breath. That was my first landing and it hadn't been bad. In fact I had got better and better all the time and the conviction was growing in me that my instructor must have been impressed with my initial showing. We climbed out and after walking a few steps in silence FO Woodham halted and turned to me.

'What's your name?' he asked.

Ah yes, here was the proof. He knew I had done well. He was interested in me.

'Herriot, sir,' I replied smartly.

For a few moments he gave me a level stare. 'Well, Herriot,' he murmured, 'that was bloody awful.'

He turned and left me. I gazed down at my feet in their big sheepskin boots. Yes, the uniform was different, but things hadn't changed all that much.

2

'Takes all kinds, doesn't it, chum?'

The airman grinned at me across the flight hut table. We had been listening to a monologue from a third man who had just left us after telling us what he intended to do after gaining his wings. The impression he left was that he was almost going to win the war on his own.

There were certainly all kinds in the RAF and this 'line shooting' was a common phenomenon when different types were thrown together.

There were all kinds of animals, too. Many people think my

farm patients are all the same, but cows, pigs, sheep and horses can be moody, placid, vicious, docile, spiteful, loving.

There was one particular pig called Gertrude, but before I come to her I must start with Mr Barge.

Nowadays the young men from the pharmaceutical companies who call on veterinary surgeons are referred to as 'reps', but nobody would have dreamed of applying such a term to Mr Barge. He was definitely a 'representative' of Cargill and Sons, Manufacturers of Fine Chemicals since 1850, and he was so old that he might have been in on the beginning.

It was a frosty morning in late winter when I opened the front door at Skeldale House and saw Mr Barge standing on the front step. He raised his black homburg a few inches above the sparse strands of silver hair and his pink features relaxed into a smile of gentle benevolence. He had always treated me as a favourite son and I took it as a compliment because he was a man of immense prestige.

'Mr Herriot,' he murmured, and bowed slightly. The bow was rich in dignity and matched the dark morning coat, striped trousers and shiny leather briefcase.

'Please come in, Mr Barge,' I said, and ushered him into the house.

He always called at midday and stayed for lunch. My young boss, Siegfried Farnon, a man not easily overawed, invariably treated him with deference and in fact the visit was something of a state occasion.

The modern rep breezes in, chats briefly about blood levels of antibiotics and steroids, says a word or two about bulk discounts, drops a few data sheets on the desk and hurries away. In a way I feel rather sorry for these young men because, with a few exceptions, they are all selling the same things.

Mr Barge, on the other hand, like all his contemporaries, carried a thick catalogue of exotic remedies, each one peculiar to its own firm.

Siegfried pulled out the chair at the head of the dining table. 'Come and sit here, Mr Barge.'

'You are very kind.' The old gentleman inclined his head slightly and took his place.

As usual there was no reference to business during the meal

and it wasn't until the coffee appeared that Mr Barge dropped his brochure carelessly on the table as though this part of the visit was an unimportant afterthought.

Siegfried and I browsed through the pages, savouring the exciting whiff of witchcraft which has been blown from our profession by the wind of science. At intervals my boss placed an order.

'I think we'd better have a couple of dozen electuaries, Mr Barge.'

'Thank you so much.' The old gentleman flipped open a leather-bound notebook and made an entry with a silver pencil.

'And we're getting a bit low on fever drinks, aren't we, James ?' Siegfried glanced round at me. 'Yes, we'll need a gross of them if you please.'

'I am most grateful,' Mr Barge breathed, noting that down, too.

My employer murmured his requests as he riffled through the catalogue. A Winchester of spirits of nitre and another of formalin, castration clams, triple bromide, Stockholm tar – all the things we never use now – and Mr Barge responded gravely to each with 'I do thank you' or 'Thank you indeed,' and a flourish of his silver pencil.

Finally Siegfried lay back in his chair. 'Well now, Mr Barge, I think that's it – unless you have anything new.'

'As it happens, my dear Mr Farnon, we have.' The eyes in the pink face twinkled. 'I can offer you our latest product, "Soothitt", an admirable sedative.'

In an instant Siegfried and I were all attention. Every animal doctor is keenly interested in sedatives. Anything which makes our patients more amenable is a blessing. Mr Barge extolled the unique properties of Soothitt and we probed for further information.

'How about unmaternal sows ?' I asked. 'You know – the kind which savage their young. I don't suppose it's any good for that ?'

'My dear young sir,' Mr Barge gave me the kind of sorrowing smile a bishop might bestow on an erring curate, 'Soothitt is a specific for this condition. A single injection to a farrowing sow and you will have no problems.'

'That's great,' I said. 'And does it have any effect on car sickness in dogs ?'

The noble old features lit up with quiet triumph. 'Another classical indication, Mr Herriot. Soothitt comes in tablet form for that very purpose.'

'Splendid.' Siegfried drained his cup and stood up. 'Better send us a good supply then. And if you will excuse us, we must start the afternoon round, Mr Barge. Thank you so much for calling.'

We all shook hands, Mr Barge raised his homburg again on the front step and another gracious occasion was over.

Within a week the new supplies from Cargill and Sons arrived. Medicines were always sent in tea chests in those days and as I prised open the wooden lid I looked with interest at the beautifully packed phials and tablets of Soothitt. And it seemed uncanny that I had a call for the new product immediately.

That same day one of the town's bank managers, Mr Ronald Beresford, called to see me.

'Mr Herriot,' he said. 'As you know I have worked here for several years but I have been offered the managership of a bigger branch down south and I leave tomorrow for Portsmouth.' From his gaunt height he looked down at me with the unsmiling gaze which was characteristic of him.

'Portsmouth! Gosh, that's a long way.'

'Yes, it is – about three hundred miles. And I have a problem.'

'Really?'

'I have, I fear. I recently purchased a six-month-old cocker spaniel and he is an excellent little animal but for the fact that he behaves peculiarly in the car.'

'In what way?'

He hesitated. 'Well, he's outside now. If you've got a minute to spare I could demonstrate.'

'Of course,' I said. 'I'll come with you now.'

We went out to the car. His wife was in the passenger seat, as fat as her husband was thin, but with the same severe unbending manner. She nodded at me coldly but the attractive little animal on her lap gave me an enthusiastic welcome.

I stroked the long silky ears. 'He's a nice little fellow.'

Mr Beresford gave me a sidelong glance. 'Yes, his name is Coco and he really is quite charming. It's only when the engine is running that the trouble begins.'

I got in the back, he pressed the starter and we set off. And I saw immediately what he meant. The spaniel stiffened and raised his head till his nose pointed at the roof. He formed his lips into a cone and emitted a series of high-pitched howls.

'Hooo, hooo, hooo, hooo,' wailed Coco.

It really startled me because I had never heard anything quite like it. I don't know whether it was the perfectly even spacing of the hoots, their piercing, jarring quality, or the fact that they never stopped which drove the sound deep into my brain, but my head was singing after a two-minute circuit of the town. I was vastly relieved when we drew up again outside the surgery.

Mr Beresford switched off the engine and it was as though he had switched off the noise, too, because the little animal relaxed instantly and began to lick my hand.

'Yes,' I said. 'You have a problem without a doubt.'

He pulled nervously at his tie. 'And it gets louder the longer you drive. Let me take you a bit further round and . . .'

'No-no, no-no,' I put in hastily. 'That won't be necessary. I can see exactly how you are placed. But you say you haven't had Coco for long. He isn't much more than a pup. I'm sure he'll get used to the car in time.'

'Very possibly he will.' Mr Beresford's voice was taut with apprehension. 'But I'm thinking of tomorrow. I've got to drive all the way to Portsmouth with my wife and this dog and I've tried car sickness tablets without result.'

A full day with that appalling din was unthinkable but at that moment the image of Mr Barge rose before me. He had sprouted wings and floated in front of my eyes like an elderly guardian angel. What an incredible piece of luck!

'As it happens,' I said with a reassuring smile, 'there is something new for this sort of thing, and by coincidence we have just received a batch of it today. Come in and I'll fix you up.'

'Well, thank heavens for that.' Mr Beresford examined the box of tablets, 'I just give one, half an hour before the journey, and all will be well?'

'That's the idea,' I replied cheerfully. 'I've given you a few extra for future journeys.'

'I am most grateful, you've taken a great load off my mind.' He went out to the car and I watched as he started the engine. As if in response to a signal the little brown head on the back seat went up and the lips pursed.

'Hooo, hooo, hooo, hooo,' Coco yowled, and his master shot me a despairing look as he drove away.

I stood on the steps for some time, listening incredulously. Many people in Darrowby didn't like Mr Beresford very much, probably because of his cold manner, but I felt he wasn't a bad chap and he certainly had my sympathy. Long after the car had disappeared round the corner of Trengate I could still hear Coco.

'Hooo, hooo, hooo, hooo.'

About seven o'clock that evening I had a phone call from Will Hollin.

'Gertrude's started farrowin'!' he said urgently. 'And she's tryin' to worry her pigs!'

It was bad news. Sows occasionally attacked their piglets after birth and in fact would kill them if they were not removed from their reach. And of course it meant that suckling was impossible.

It was a tricky problem at any time but particularly so in this case because Gertrude was a pedigree sow – an expensive animal Will Hollin had bought to improve his strain of pigs.

'How many has she had?' I asked.

'Four – and she's gone for every one.' His voice was tense.

It was then I remembered Soothitt and again I blessed the coming of Mr Barge.

I smiled into the receiver. 'There's a new product I can use, Mr Hollin. Just arrived today. I'll be right out.'

I trotted through to the dispensary, opened the box of phials and had a quick read at the enclosed pamphlet. Ah yes, there it was. 'Ten cc intramuscularly and the sow will accept the piglets within twenty minutes.'

It wasn't a long drive to the Hollin farm but as I sped through the darkness I could discern the workings of fate in the day's events. The Soothitt had arrived this morning and right away I had two urgent calls for it. There was no doubt Mr Barge had been sent for a purpose – living proof, perhaps, that everything in our lives is preordained. It gave me a prickling at the back of my neck to think about it.

I could hardly wait to get the injection into the sow and climbed eagerly into the pen. Gertrude didn't appreciate having a needle rammed into her thigh and she swung round on me with an explosive bark. But I got the ten cc in before making my escape.

'We just wait twenty minutes, then ?' Will Hollin leaned on the rail and looked down anxiously at his pig. He was a hardworking smallholder in his fifties and I knew this meant a lot to him.

I was about to make a comforting reply when Gertrude popped out another pink, squirming piglet. The farmer leaned over and gently nudged the little creature towards the udder as the sow lay on her side, but as soon as the nose made contact with the teat the big pig was up in a flash, all growls and yellow teeth.

He snatched the piglet away quickly and deposited it with the others in a tall cardboard box. 'Well, you see how it is, Mr Herriot.'

'I certainly do. How many have you got in there now ?'

'There's six. And they're grand pigs, too.'

I peered into the box at the little animals. They all had the classical long-bodied shape. 'Yes, they are. And she looks as though she has a lot more in her yet.'

The farmer nodded and we waited.

It seemed to take a long time for the twenty minutes to pass but finally I lifted a couple of piglets and clambered into the pen. I was about to put them to the sow when one of them squealed. Gertrude rushed across with a ferocious roar, mouth gaping, and I leaped to safety with an agility which surprised me.

'She don't look very sleepy,' Mr Hollin said.

'No . . . no . . . she doesn't, does she ? Maybe we'd better wait a bit longer.'

We gave her another ten minutes and tried again with the same result. I injected a further ten cc of the Soothitt, then about an hour later a third one. By nine o'clock Gertrude had produced fifteen beautiful young pigs and had chased me and her family from the pen six times. She was, if anything, livelier and fiercer than when I started.

'Well, she's cleansed,' Mr Hollin said gloomily. 'So it looks like she's finished.' He gazed, sad-faced, into the box. 'And now I've got fifteen pigs to rear without their mother's milk. I could lose all this lot.'

'Nay, nay.' The voice came from the open doorway. 'You won't lose 'em.'

I looked round. It was Grandad Hollin, his puckish features set in their customary smile. He marched to the pen and poked Gertrude's ribs with his stick.

She responded with a snarl and a malignant glare and the old man's smile grew broader.

'Ah'll soon fettle the awd beggar,' he said.

'Fettle her?' I shifted my feet uncomfortably. 'What do you mean?'

'Why, she just wants quietin', tha knaws.'

I took a long breath. 'Yes, Mr Hollin, that's exactly what I've been trying to do.'

'Aye, but you're not doin' it the right way, young man.'

I looked at him narrowly. The know-all with his liberal advice in a difficult situation is a familiar figure most veterinary surgeons have to tolerate, but in Grandad Hollin's case I didn't feel the usual irritation. I liked him. He was a nice man, the head of a fine family. Will was the eldest of his four sons and he had several farmer grandsons in the district.

Anyway, I had failed miserably. I was in no position to be uppity.

'Well, I've given her the latest injection,' I mumbled.

He shook his head. 'She don't want injections, she wants beer.'

'Eh?'

'Beer, young man. A drop o' good ale.' He turned to his son. 'Hasta got a clean bucket, Will, lad?'

'Aye, there's a new-scalded one in t'milk house.'

'Right, ah'll slip down to the pub. Won't be long.' Grandad swung on his heel and strode briskly into the night. He must have been around eighty but from the back he looked like a twenty-five-year-old – upright, square-shouldered, jaunty.

Will Hollin and I didn't have much to say to each other. He was sunk in disappointment and I was awash with shame. It was a relief when Grandad returned bearing an enamel bucket brimming with brown liquid.

'By gaw,' he chuckled. 'You should've seen their faces down at t'Wagon and Horses. Reckon they've never heard of a two-gallon order afore.'

I gaped at him. 'You've got two gallons of beer?'

'That's right, young man, and she'll need it all.' He turned again to his son. 'She hasn't had a drink for a bit, has she, Will ?'

'Naw, I was goin' to give her some water when she'd finished piggin' but I haven't done it yet.'

Grandad poised his bucket. 'She'll be nice and thirsty, then.' He leaned over the rail and sent a dark cascade frothing into the empty trough.

Gertrude ambled moodily across and sniffed at the strange fluid. After some hesitation she dipped her snout and tried a tentative swallow, and within seconds the building echoed with a busy slobbering.

'By heck, she likes it!' Will exclaimed.

'She should,' Grandad murmured wistfully. 'It's John Smith's best bitter.'

It took the sow a surprisingly short time to consume the two gallons and when she had finished she licked out every corner of the trough before turning away. She showed no inclination to return to her straw bed but began to saunter round the pen. Now and then she stopped at the trough to check that there was no more beer in it and from time to time she looked up at the three faces overhanging the timber walls.

On one of these occasions I caught her eye and saw with a sense of disbelief that the previously baleful little orb now registered only a gentle benevolence. In fact with a little effort I could have imagined she was smiling.

As the minutes passed her perambulations became increasingly erratic. There were times when she stumbled and almost fell and finally with an unmistakeable hiccup she flopped on the straw and rolled on to her side.

Grandad regarded her expressionlessly for a few moments, whistling tunelessly, then he reached out again and pushed his stick against the fleshy thigh, but the only response he received from the motionless animal was a soft grunt of pleasure.

Gertrude was stoned to the wide.

The old man gestured towards the cardboard box. 'Put the little 'uns in now.'

Will went into the pen with a wriggling armful, then another, and like all newborn creatures they didn't have to be told what to do. Fifteen ravenous little mouths fastened on to the teats and with mixed feelings I gazed at the sight which I had hoped to bring about with my modern veterinary skill, the long pink row filling their tiny stomachs with the life-giving fluid.

Well, I had fallen down on the job and an octogenarian farmer had wiped my eye with two gallons of strong ale. I didn't feel great.

Sheepishly I closed the box of Soothitt phials and was beating an unobtrusive retreat to my car when Will Hollin called after me.

'Come in and have a cup o' coffee afore you go, Mr Herriot.' His voice was friendly, with nothing to suggest that I had made no useful contribution all evening.

I made my way into the kitchen and as I went over to the table Will dug me in the ribs.

'Hey, look at this.' He held out the bucket in which a quantity of the good beer still sloshed around the bottom. 'There's summat better than coffee 'ere – enough for a couple of good drinks. I'll get two glasses.'

He was fumbling in the dresser when Grandad walked in. The old man hung his hat and stick on a hook on the wall and rubbed his hands.

'Tha can get another glass out, Will,' he said. 'Remember ah did the pourin' and ah left enough for three.'

Next morning I might have been inclined to dwell despondently on my chastening experience but I had a pre-breakfast call to a cow with a prolapsed uterus and there is nothing like an hour of feverish activity to rid the mind of brooding.

It was 8 a.m. when I drove back into Darrowby and I pulled in to the market place petrol station which was just opening. With a pleasantly blank mind I was watching Bob Cooper running the petrol in the tank when I heard the sound in the distance.

'Hooo, hooo, hooo, hooo.'

Tremblingly I scanned the square. There was no other vehicle in sight but the dread ululation approached inexorably until Mr Beresford's car rounded the far corner, heading my way.

I shrank behind a petrol pump but it was of no avail. I had been spotted and the car bumped over the strip of cobbles before screeching to a halt beside me.

'Hooo, hooo, hooo, hooo.' At close quarters the noise was insupportable.

I peeped round the pump and into the bulging eyes of the bank manager as he lowered his window. He switched off the engine and Coco stopped his howling and gave me a friendly wag through the glass.

His master, however, did not look at all friendly.

'Good morning, Mr Herriot,' he said, grim-faced.

'Good morning,' I replied hoarsely, then working up a smile I bent at the window. 'And good morning to you, Mrs Beresford.'

The lady withered me with a look and was about to speak when her husband went on.

'I administered one of the wonderful new tablets early this morning on your advice.' His chin quivered slightly.

'Oh, yes . . . ?'

'Yes, I did, and it had no effect, so I gave him another.' He paused. 'Since this produced a similar result I tried a third and a fourth.'

I swallowed. 'Really . . . ?'

'Indeed.' He gave me a cold stare. 'So I am driven to the conclusion that the tablets are useless.'

'Well . . . er . . . it certainly does look . . .'

He held up a hand. 'I cannot listen to explanations. I have already wasted enough time and there are three hundred miles' driving in front of me.'

'I'm truly sorry . . .' I began, but he was already closing the window. He started the engine and Coco froze immediately into his miniature wolf position, nose high, lips puckered into a small circle. I watched the car roll across the square and turn out of sight on the road to the south. For quite a while after it had gone I could still hear Coco.

'Hooo, hooo, hooo, hooo.'

Feeling suddenly weak, I leaned against the pump. My heart went out to Mr Beresford. As I have said, I felt sure he was a decent man.

In fact I quite liked him, but for all that I was profoundly grateful that I would probably never see him again.

*

Our audiences with Mr Barge usually took place every three months and it was mid-June before I saw him again at the head of our luncheon table. The silvery head gleamed under the summer sunshine as he sipped his coffee and murmured politenesses. At the end of the meal he dabbed his lips with a napkin and slid his brochure unhurriedly along the table cloth.

Siegfried reached for it and asked the inevitable question. 'Anything new, Mr Barge ?'

'My dear sir.' The old gentleman's smile seemed to convey that the follies of the young, though incomprehensible to him, were still delightful. 'Cargill and Sons never send me to you without a host of new products, many of them specific, all of them efficient. I have many sovereign remedies to offer you.'

I must have uttered some sort of strangled sound because he turned and regarded me quizzically. 'Ah, Mr Herriot, did you say something, young sir ?'

I swallowed a couple of times and opened my mouth as the waves of benevolence flowed over me, but against that dignity and presence I was helpless.

'No . . . no, not really, Mr Barge,' I replied. I knew I would never be able to tell him about the Soothitt.

3

Now that we were faced with the reality of life at flying school, the ties which bound me to my fellow airmen were strengthened. We had a common aim, a common worry.

The feeling of comradeship was very like my relationship with Siegfried, and his student brother, Tristan, back in Darrowby. But there, the pressures came not from learning to fly but from the daily challenge of veterinary practice. Our existence was ruled by sudden and unexpected alarms.

Tristan, however, didn't let it get him down. He and I were sitting in the big room at Skeldale House one night when the telephone burst into strident voice.

He reached from his chair and lifted the receiver.

'Allo, plis, oo is dis?' he inquired.

He listened attentively for a few moments then shook his head. 'Naw, naw, verree sorry, but Meester Farnon no at home. Yis, yis, I tell heem when he come. Hokey dokey, bye bye.'

I looked across at him wonderingly from the other side of the fireplace as he replaced the instrument. These strange accents were only one facet of his constant determination to extract amusement from every situation. He didn't do it all the time, only when the mood was on him, but it was not unusual for farmers to say that 'some foreign feller' had answered the phone.

Tristan settled comfortably behind his *Daily Mirror* and was fumbling for a Woodbine when the ringing started again. He stretched out once more.

'Yaas, yaas, goot efening, howdy do. Vat you vant, huh?'

I could just hear a deep rumble from the other end of the line and Tristan suddenly snapped upright in his chair. His *Daily Mirror* and cigarettes slithered to the floor.

'Yes, Mr Mouht,' he said smartly. 'No, Mr Mount. Yes indeed, Mr Mount, I shall pass on your message immediately. Thank you very much, goodbye.'

He fell back in the chair and blew out his cheeks. 'That was Mr Mount.'

'So I gathered. And he certainly wiped the smile off your face, Triss.'

'Yes . . . yes . . . just a little unexpected.' He recovered his Woodbines and lit one thoughtfully.

'Quite,' I said. 'What did he ring for, anyway?'

'Oh, he has a cart horse to see tomorrow morning. Something wrong with its hind feet.'

I made a note on the pad and turned back to the young man. 'I don't know how you find the time in your hectic love life, but you're running around with that chap's daughter, aren't you?'

Tristan took the cigarette from his mouth and studied the glowing end. 'Yes, as a matter of fact I have taken Deborah Mount out a few times. Why do you ask?'

'Oh, no particular reason. Her old man seems a bit formidable, that's all.'

I could picture Mr Mount the last time I saw him. He was well named; a veritable massif of a man towering several inches over six feet. From shoulders like the great buttresses of the fell which overhung his farm rose a beetling cliff of head with craggy outcrops of jaw and cheek and brow. He had the biggest hands I have ever seen – approximately three times the size of my own.

'Oh, I don't know,' Tristan said. 'He's not a bad sort.'

'I agree, I've nothing against him.' Mr Mount was deeply religious and had the reputation of being hard but fair. 'It's just that I wouldn't like him to come up to me and ask if I was trifling with his daughter's affections.'

Tristan swallowed, and anxiety flitted briefly in his eyes. 'Oh, that's ridiculous. Deborah and I have a friendly relationship, that's all.'

'Well, I'm glad to hear it,' I said. 'I've been told her father is very protective about her and I'd hate to feel those big hands round my throat.'

Tristan gave me a cold stare. 'You're a sadistic bugger at times, Jim. Just because I occasionally enjoy a little female company . . .'

'Oh, forget it, Triss, I'm only kidding. You've nothing to worry about. When I see old Mount tomorrow I promise I won't mention that Deborah is one of your harem.' I dodged a flying cushion and went through to the dispensary to stock up for the next day's round.

But I realized next morning that my joke was barbed when I saw Mr Mount coming out of the farmhouse. For a moment his bulk filled the doorway, then he advanced with measured tread over the cobbles till he loomed over me, blocking out the sunshine, throwing a large area around me into shade.

'That young man, Tristan,' he said without preamble. 'He was speakin' a bit funny like on the phone last night. What sort of a feller is he ?'

I looked up at the great head poised above me, at the unwavering grey eyes probing into mine from beneath a bristling overhang of brow. 'Tristan ?' I answered shakily. 'Oh, he's a splendid chap. A really fine type.'

'Mmm.' The huge man continued to look at me and one bananalike finger rubbed doubtfully along his chin. 'Does he drink ?'

Mr Mount was renowned for his rigid antagonism to alcohol

and I thought it unwise to reply that Tristan was a popular and esteemed figure at most of the local hostelries.

'Oh, er—' I said. 'Hardly at all . . . in the strictest moderation . . .'

At that moment Deborah came out of the house and began to walk across the yard.

She was wearing a flowered cotton dress. About nineteen, shining golden hair falling below her shoulders, she radiated the healthy buxom beauty of the country girl. As she went by she flashed a smile at me and I had a heart-lifting glimpse of white teeth and warm brown eyes. It was in the early days before I had met Helen and I had as sharp an interest in a pretty lass as anybody. I found myself studying her legs appreciatively after she had passed.

It was then that I had an almost palpable awareness of her father's gaze upon me. I turned and saw a new expression there – a harsh disapproval which chilled me and left a deep conviction in my mind. Deborah was a little smasher all right, and she looked nice, too, but no . . . no . . . never. Tristan had more courage than I had.

Mr Mount turned away abruptly. 'This 'oss is in the stable,' he grunted.

In those late thirties the tractor had driven a lot of the draught horses from the land but most of the farmers kept a few around, perhaps because they had always worked horses and it was part of their way of life and maybe because of the sheer proud beauty of animals like the one which stood before me now.

It was a magnificent Shire gelding, standing all of eighteen hands. He was a picture of massively muscled power but when his master spoke, the great white-blazed face which turned to us was utterly docile.

The farmer slapped him on the rump. 'He's a good sort is Bobby and I think a bit about 'im. What ah noticed first was a strange smell about his hind feet and then ah had a look for meself. I've never seen owt like it.'

I bent and seized a handful of the long feathered hair behind the horse's pastern. Bobby did not resist as I lifted the huge spatulate foot and rested it on my knee. It seemed to occupy most of my lap but it was not the size which astonished me. Mr Mount had never seen owt like it and neither had I. The sole was a ragged, sodden mass with a stinking exudation oozing from the underrun horn, but what really bewildered me was the series of growths sprouting from every crevice.

They were like nightmare toadstools – long papillae with horny caps growing from the diseased surface. I had read about them in the books; they were called ergots, but I had never imagined them in such profusion. My thoughts raced as I moved behind the horse and lifted the other foot. It was just the same. Just as bad.

I had been qualified only a few months and was still trying to gain the confidence of the Darrowby farmers. This was just the sort of thing I didn't want.

'What is it?' Mr Mount asked, and again I felt that unwinking gaze piercing me.

I straightened up and rubbed my hands. 'It's canker, but a very bad case.' I knew all about the theory of the thing, in fact I was bursting with theory, but putting it into practice with this animal was a bit different.

'How are you going to cure it?' Mr Mount had an uncomfortable habit of going straight to the heart of things.

'Well, you see, all that loose horn and those growths will have to be cut away and then the surface dressed with caustic,' I replied, and it sounded easy when I said it.

'It won't get better on its own, then?'

'No, if you leave it the sole will disintegrate and the pedal bone will come through. Also the discharge will work up under the wall of the hoof and cause separation.'

The farmer nodded. 'So he'd never walk again, and that would be the end of Bobby.'

'I'm afraid so.'

'Right, then.' Mr Mount threw up his head with a decisive gesture. 'When are you going to do it?'

It was a nasty question, because I was preoccupied at that moment not so much with when I would do it but how I would do it.

'Well now, let's see,' I said huskily. 'Would it be . . .' The farmer broke in. 'We're busy hay-makin' all this week, and you'll be wantin' some men to help you. How about Monday next week?'

A wave of relief surged through me. Thank heavens he hadn't said tomorrow. I had a bit of time to think now.

'Very well, Mr Mount. That suits me fine. Don't feed him on the Sunday because he'll have to have an anaesthetic.'

Driving from the farm, a sense of doom oppressed me. Was I going to ruin that beautiful animal in my ignorance? Canker of the foot was unpleasant at any time and was not uncommon in the days of the draught horse, but this was something way out of the ordinary. No doubt many of my contemporaries have seen feet like Bobby's, but to the modern young veterinary surgeon it must be like a page from an ancient manual of farriery.

As is my wont when I have a worrying case I started mulling it over right away. As I drove, I rehearsed various procedures. Would that enormous horse go down with a chloroform muzzle? Or would I have to collect all Mr Mount's men and rope him and pull him down? But it would be like trying to pull down St Paul's Cathedral. And then how long would it take me to hack away all that horn – all those dreadful vegetations?

Within ten minutes my palms were sweating and I was tempted to throw the whole lot over to Siegfried. But I was restrained by the knowledge that I had to establish myself not only with the farmers but with my new boss. He wasn't going to think much of an assistant who couldn't handle a thing on his own.

I did what I usually did when I was worried: drove off the un-fenced road, got out of the car and followed a track across the moor. The track wound beneath the brow of the fell which over-looked the Mount farm and when I had left the road far behind I flopped on the grass and looked down on the sunlit valley floor a thousand feet below.

In most places you could hear something – the call of a bird, a car in the distance – but here there was a silence which was abso-lute, except when the wind sighed over the hilltop, rustling the bracken around me.

The farm lay in one of the soft places in a harsh countryside; lush flat fields where cattle grazed in comfort and the cut hay lay in long even swathes.

It was a placid scene, but it was up here in the airy heights that you found true serenity. Peace dwelt here in the high moorland, stealing across the empty miles, breathing from the silence and the tufted grass and the black, peaty earth.

The heady fragrance of the hay rose in the warm summer air and as always I felt my troubles dissolving. Even now, after all the years, I still count myself lucky that I can so often find tranquility of mind in the high places.

As I rose to go I was filled with a calm resolve. I would do the job somehow. Surely I could manage the thing without troubling Siegfried.

In any case Siegfried had other things on his mind when I met him over the lunch table.

'I looked in at Granville Bennett's surgery at Hartington this morning,' he said, helping himself to some new potatoes which had been picked that morning from the garden. 'And I must say I was very impressed with his waiting room. All those magazines. I know we don't have the numbers to cater for, but there's often a lot of farmers in there.' He poured gravy on to a corner of his plate. 'Tristan, I'll give you the job. Slip round to Garlow's and order a few suitable things to be delivered every week, will you ?'

'Okay,' his student brother replied. 'I'll do it this afternoon.'

'Splendid.' Siegfried chewed happily. 'We must keep progressing in every way. Do have some more of these potatoes, James, they really are very good.'

Tristan went into action right away and within two days the table and shelves in our waiting room carried a tasteful selection of periodicals. The *Illustrated London News*, *Farmer's Weekly*, *The Farmer and Stockbreeder*, *Punch*. But as usual he had to embroider the situation.

'Look at this, Jim,' he whispered one afternoon, guiding me through the door. 'I've been having a little harmless sport.'

'What do you mean ?' I looked around me uncomprehendingly.

Tristan said nothing, but pointed to one of the shelves. There, among the innocent journals was a German naturist magazine displaying a startling frontispiece of full frontal nudity. Even in these permissive days it would have caused a raised eyebrow but in rural Yorkshire in the thirties it was cataclysmic.

'Where the devil did you get this ?' I gasped, leafing through it hurriedly. It was just the same inside. 'And what's the idea, anyway?'

Tristan repressed a giggle. 'A fellow at college gave it to me. And it's rather a lark to sneak in quietly and find some solid citizen having a peek when he thinks nobody's looking. I've had some very successful incursions. My best bags so far have been a town councillor, a Justice of the Peace and a lay preacher.'

I shook my head. 'I think you're sticking your neck out. What if Siegfried comes across it?'

'No fear of that,' he said. 'He rarely comes in here and he's always in too much of a hurry. Anyway, it's well out of the way.'

I shrugged. Tristan had been blessed with an agile intelligence which I envied, but so much of it was misapplied. However, at the moment I hadn't time for his tricks. My mind was feverishly preoccupied.

Mentally I had cast that horse by innumerable methods and operated on his feet a thousand times by night and day. In daylight, riding around in the car, it wasn't so bad, but the operations I carried out in bed were truly bizarre. All the time I had the feeling that something was wrong, that there was some fatal flaw in the picture of myself carving away those hideous growths in one session. Finally I buried my pride.

'Siegfried,' I said, one afternoon when the practice was slack. 'I have rather a weird horse case.'

My boss's eyes glinted and the mouth beneath the small sandy moustache crooked into a smile. The word 'horse' usually had this effect.

'Really, James? Tell me.'

I told him.

'Yes . . . yes . . .' he murmured. 'Maybe we'd better have a look together.'

The Mount farm was deserted when we arrived. Everybody was in the hayfields working frantically while the sunshine lasted.

'Where is he?' Siegfried asked.

'In here.' I led the way to the stable.

My boss lifted a hind foot and whistled softly. Then he moved round and examined the other one. For a full minute he gazed down at the obscene fungi thrusting from the tattered stinking horn. When he stood up he looked at me expressionlessly.

It was a few seconds before he spoke. 'And you were just going to pop round here on Monday, tip this big fellow on to the grass and do the job?'

'Yes,' I replied. 'That was the idea.'

A strange smile spread over my employer's face. It held something of wonder, sympathy, amusement and a tinge of admiration. Finally he laughed and shook his head.

'Ah, the innocence of youth,' he murmured.

'What do you mean?' After all, I was only six years younger than Siegfried.

He came over and patted my shoulder. 'I'm not mocking you, James. This is the worst case of canker I've ever seen and I've seen a few.'

'You mean I couldn't do it at one go?'

'That's exactly what I mean. There's six weeks' work here, James.'

'Six weeks...?'

'Yes, and there'll be three men involved. We'll have to get this horse into one of the loose boxes at Skeldale House and then the two of us plus a blacksmith will have a go at him. After that his feet will have to be dressed every day in the stocks.'

'I see.'

'Yes, yes.' Siegfried was warming to his subject. 'We'll use the strongest caustic – nitric acid – and he'll be shod with special shoes with a metal plate to exert pressure on the sole.' He stopped, probably because I was beginning to look bewildered, then he continued in a gentler tone. 'Believe me, James, all this is necessary. The alternative is to shoot a fine horse, because he can't go on much longer than this.'

I looked at Bobby, at the white face again turned towards us. The thought of a bullet entering that noble head was unbearable.

'All right, whatever you say, Siegfried,' I mumbled, and just then Mr Mount's vast bulk darkened the entrance to the stable.

'Ah, good afternoon to you, Mr Mount,' my boss said. 'I hope you're getting a good crop of hay.'

'Aye, thank ye, Mr Farnon. We're doing very nicely. We've been lucky with the weather.' The big man looked curiously from one of us to the other, and Siegfried went on quickly.

'Mr Herriot asked me to come and look at your horse. He's been thinking the matter over and has decided that it would be better to hospitalize him at our place for a few weeks. I must say I agree with him. It's a very bad case and the chances of a permanent cure would be increased.'

Bless you, Siegfried, I thought. I had expected to emerge from this meeting as the number one chump, but all was suddenly well. I congratulated myself, not for the first time, on having an employer who never let me down.

Mr Mount took off his hat and drew a forearm across his sweating brow. 'Aye well, if that's what you think, both of ye, we'd better do it. Ah want the best for Bobby. He's a favourite o' mine.'

'Yes, he's a grand sort, Mr Mount.' Siegfried went round the big animal, patting and stroking him, then as we walked back to the car he kept up an effortless conversation with the farmer. I had always found it difficult to speak to this formidable man, but in my colleague's presence he became quite chatty. In fact there were one or two occasions when he almost smiled.

Bobby came into the yard at Skeldale House the following day and when I saw the amount of sheer hard labour which the operation entailed I realized the utter impossibility of a single man doing it at one go.

Pat Jenner, the blacksmith, with his full tool kit was pressed into service and between us, taking it in turns, we removed all the vegetations and diseased tissue, leaving only healthy horn. Siegfried applied the acid to cauterize the area, then packed the sole with twists of tow which were held in place by the metal plate Pat had made to fit under the shoe. This pressure from the tow was essential to effect a cure.

After a week I was doing the daily dressings myself. This was when I began to appreciate the value of the stocks with their massive timbers sunk deep into the cobbles of the yard. It made everything so much easier when I was able to lead Bobby into the stocks, pull up a foot and make it fast in any position I wished.

Some days Pat Jenner came in to check on the shoes, and he and I were busy in the yard when I heard the familiar rattle of my little Austin in the back lane. The big double doors were open and I looked up as the car turned in and drew alongside us. Pat looked, too, and his eyes popped.

'Bloody 'ell!' he exclaimed, and I couldn't blame him, because the car had no driver. At least it looked that way since there was nobody in the seat as it swung in from the lane.

A driverless car in motion is quite a sight, and Pat gaped open-mouthed for a few seconds. Then just as I was about to explain, Tristan shot up from the floor with a piercing cry.

'Hi there!' he shrieked.

Pat dropped his hammer and backed away. 'God 'elp us!' he breathed.

I was unaffected by the performance because it was old stuff to me. Whenever I was in the yard and a call came in, Tristan would drive my car round from the front street and this happened so many times that inevitably he grew bored and tried to find a less orthodox method.

After a bit of practice he mastered the driverless technique. He crouched on the floor with a foot on the accelerator and one hand on the wheel and nearly frightened the life out of me the first time he did it. But I was used to it now, and blasé.

Within a few days I was able to observe another of Tristan's little jokes. As I turned the corner of the passage at Skeldale House I found him lurking by the waiting-room door which was slightly ajar.

'I think I've got a victim in there,' he whispered. 'Let's see what happens.' He gently pushed the door and tiptoed inside.

As I peeped through the crack I could see that he had indeed scored a success. A man was standing there with his back to him and he was poring over the nudist magazine with greatest absorption. As he slowly turned the pages his enthralment showed in the way he frequently moved the pictures towards the light from the french window, inclining his head this way and that to take in all the angles. He looked as though he would have been happy to spend all day there but when he heard Tristan's exquisitely timed cough he dropped the magazine as thought it was white hot, snatched hurriedly at the *Farmer's Weekly* and swung round.

That was when Tristan's victory went flat. It was Mr Mount.

The huge farmer loomed over him for a few seconds and the deep bass rumble came from between clenched teeth.

'It's you, is it?' He glanced quickly from the young man to the embarrassing magazine and back again and the eyes in the craggy face narrowed dangerously.

'Yes . . . yes . . . yes, Mr Mount,' Tristan replied unsteadily. 'And how are you, Mr Mount?'

'Ah'm awright.'

'Good . . . good . . . splendid.' Tristan backed away a few steps. 'And how is Deborah?'

The eyes beneath the sprouting bristles drew in further. 'She's awright.'

There was a silence which lingered interminably and I felt for my young friend. It was not a merry meeting.

At last he managed to work up a sickly smile. 'Ah well, yes, er . . . and what can we do for you, Mr Mount?'

'Ah've come to see me 'oss.'

'Yes indeed, of course, certainly. I believe Mr Herriot is just outside the room.'

I led the big man down the long garden into the yard. His encounter with Tristan had clearly failed to improve his opinion of the young man and he glowered as I opened the loose box.

But his expression softened when he saw Bobby eating hay contentedly. He went in and patted the arching neck. 'How's he goin' on then?'

'Oh, very well.' I lifted a hind foot and showed him the metal plate. 'I can take this off for you if you like.'

'Nay, nay, ah don't want to disturb the job. As long as all's well, that's all ah want to know.'

The dressings went on for a few more weeks till finally Siegfried was satisfied that the last remnants of the disease had been extirpated. Then he telephoned for Mr Mount to collect his horse the following morning.

It is always nice to be in on a little triumph, and I looked over my boss's shoulder as he lifted Bobby's feet and displayed the finished job to the owner. The necrotic jumble on the soles had been replaced by a clean, smooth surface with no sign of moisture anywhere.

Mr Mount was not enthusiastic by nature but he was obviously impressed. He nodded his head rapidly several times. 'Well now, that's champion. I'm right capped wi' that.'

Siegfried lowered the foot to the ground and straightened with a pleased smile. There was a general air of bonhomie in the yard, and then I heard my car in the back lane.

I felt a sudden tingle of apprehension. Oh no, Tristan, not this time, please. You don't know ... My toes curled as I waited but I realized all was lost when the car turned in through the double doors. It had no driver.

With a dreadful feeling of imminent catastrophe I watched as it stopped within a few feet of Siegfried and Mr Mount who were staring at it in disbelief.

Nothing happened for a few seconds, then without warning Tristan catapulted like a jack-in-the-box into the open window.

'Yippeeee!' he screeched, but his happy grin froze as he found himself gazing into the faces of his brother and Mr Mount. Siegfried's expression of exasperation was familiar to me, but the farmer's was infinitely more menacing. The eyes in the stony visage were mere slits, the jaw jutted, the great tangle of eyebrows bristled fiercely. There was no doubt he had finally made up his mind about Tristan.

I felt the young man had suffered enough, and I kept off the subject for a week or two afterwards, but we were sitting in the big room at Skeldale House when he mentioned casually that he wouldn't be taking Deborah out any more.

'Seems her father has forbidden it,' he said.

I shrugged in sympathy, but said nothing. After all, it had been an ill-starred romance from the beginning.

4

'Circuits and Bumps' they called it. Taking off, circling the field and landing, over and over and over. After an hour of it with FO Woodham in full voice I had had enough and it was a blessed relief when we climbed out at the end.

As my instructor walked away, one of his fellow officers

strolled by his side. 'How are you getting on with that chap, Woody ?' he asked, smiling.

FO Woodham did not pause in his stride or turn his head. 'Oh, God!' he said with a hollow groan, and that was all.

I knew I wasn't meant to hear the words but they bit deep. My spirits did not rise till I entered the barrack hut and was greeted by the cheerful voices of my fellow airmen.

'Hello, Jim!' 'How's it going, Jim ?' The words were like balm.

I looked around at the young men sprawled on their beds, reading or smoking and I realized that I needed them and their friendship.

Animals are the same. They need friends. Have you ever watched two animals in a field ? They may be different species – a pony and a sheep – but they hang together. This comradeship between animals has always fascinated me, and I often think of Jack Sanders's two dogs as a perfect example of mutual devotion.

One of them was called Jingo and as I injected the local anaesthetic alongside the barbed wire tear in his skin the powerful bull terrier whimpered just once. Then he decided to resign himself to his fate and looked stolidly to the front as I depressed the plunger.

Meanwhile his inseparable friend, Skipper the corgi, gnawed gently at Jingo's hind leg. It was odd to see two dogs on the table at once, but I knew the relationship between them and made no comment as their master hoisted them both up.

After I had infiltrated the area around the wound I began to stitch and Jingo relaxed noticeably when he found that he could feel nothing.

'Maybe this'll teach you to avoid barbed wire fences in future, Jing,' I said.

Jack Sanders laughed. 'I doubt if it will, Mr Herriot. I thought the coast was clear when I took him down the lane this morning, but he spotted a dog on the other side of the fence and he was through like a bullet. Fortunately it was a greyhound and he couldn't catch it.'

'You're a regular terror, Jing.' I patted my patient, and the big Roman-nosed face turned to me with an ear-to-ear grin and at the other end the tail whipped delightedly.

'Yes, it's amazing, isn't it ?' his master said. 'He's always looking for a fight, yet people and children can do anything with him. He's the best natured dog in the world.'

I finished stitching and dropped the suture needle into a kidney dish on the trolley. 'Well, you've got to remember that the bull terrier is the original English fighting dog and Jing is only obeying an age-old instinct.'

'Oh, I realize that. I'll just have to go on scanning the horizon every time I let him off the lead. No dog is safe from him.'

'Except this one, Jack.' I laughed and pointed to the little corgi who had tired of his companion's leg and was now chewing his ear.

'Yes, isn't it marvellous. I think he could bite Jing's ear off without reprisal.'

It was indeed rather wonderful. The corgi was eleven years old and beginning to show his age in stiffness of movement and impairment of sight, while the bull terrier was only three, at the height of his strength and power. A squat, barrel-chested bundle of bone and muscle, he was a formidable animal. But when the ear-chewing became too violent, all he did was turn and gently engulf Skipper's head in his huge jaws till the little animal desisted. Those jaws could be as merciless as a steel trap but they held the tiny head in a loving embrace.

Ten days later their master brought both dogs back to the surgery for the removal of the stitches. He looked worried as he lifted the animals on to the table.

'Jingo isn't at all well, Mr Herriot,' he said. 'He's been off his food for a couple of days and he looks miserable. Could that wound make him ill if it turned septic?'

'Yes it could, of course.' I looked down anxiously at the area of the flank where I had stitched, and my fingers explored the long scar. 'But there's not the slightest sign of infection here. No swelling, no pain. He's healed beautifully.'

I stepped back and looked at the bull terrier. He was strangely disconsolate, tail tucked down, eyes gazing ahead with total lack of interest. Not even the busy nibbling of his friend at one of his paws relieved his apathy.

Clearly Skipper didn't like being ignored in this fashion. He transferred his operations to the front end and started on the big dog's ear. As his efforts still went unnoticed he began to chew and tug harder, dragging the massive head down to one side, but as far as Jingo was concerned he might as well not have been there.

'Hey, that's enough, Skipper,' I said. 'Jing isn't in the mood for rough stuff today.' I lifted him gently to the floor where he paced indignantly around the table legs.

I examined the bull terrier thoroughly and the only significant finding was an elevated temperature.

'It's a hundred and five, Jack. He's very ill, there's no doubt about that.'

'But what's the matter with him?'

'With a high fever like that he must have some acute infection. But at the moment it's difficult to pinpoint.' I reached out and stroked the broad skull, running my fingers over the curving white face as my thoughts raced.

For an instant the tail twitched between his hocks and the friendly eyes rolled round to me and then to his master. It was that movement of the eyes which seized my whole attention. I quickly raised the upper lid. The conjunctiva appeared to be a normal pink, but in the smooth white sclera I could discern the faintest tinge of yellow.

'He's got jaundice,' I said. 'Have you noticed anything peculiar about his urine?'

Jack Sanders nodded. 'Yes, now you mention it. I saw him cock his leg in the garden and his water looked a bit dark.'

'Those are bile pigments.' I gently squeezed the abdomen and the dog winced slightly. 'Yes, he's definitely tender in there.'

'Jaundice?' His master stared at me across the table. 'Where would he get that?'

I rubbed my chin. 'Well, when I see a dog like this I think firstly of two things – phosphorus poisoning and leptospirosis. In view of the high temperature I go for the leptospirosis.'

'Would he catch it from another dog?'

'Possibly, but more likely from rats. Does he come into contact with any rats?'

'Yes, now and then. There's a lot of them in an old hen house at the foot of the lane and Jing sometimes gets in there after them.'

43

'Well, that's it.' I shrugged. 'I don't think we need to look any further for the cause.'

He nodded slowly. 'Anyway, it's something to know what's wrong with him. Now you can set about putting him right.'

I looked at him for a moment in silence. It wasn't like that at all. I didn't want to upset him, but on the other hand he was a highly intelligent and sensible man in his forties, a teacher at the local school. I felt I had to tell him the whole truth.

'Jack,' I said. 'This is a terrible condition to treat. If there's one thing I hate to see it's a jaundiced dog.'

'You mean it's serious ?'

'I'm afraid so. In fact the mortality rate is very high.'

I felt for him when I saw the sudden pain and concern in his face, but a warning now was better than a shock later, because I knew that Jingo could be dead within a few days. Even now, thirty years later, I quail when I see that yellowish discoloration in a dog's eyes. Penicillin and other antibiotics have some effect against the causal organism of leptospirosis but the disease is still very often fatal.

'I see . . . I see . . .' He was collecting his thoughts. 'But surely you can do something ?'

'Yes, yes, of course,' I said briskly. 'I'm going to give him a big shot of antileptospiral serum and some medicine to administer by the mouth. It isn't completely hopeless.'

I injected the serum in the knowledge that it didn't have much effect at this stage, but I had nothing else to offer. I gave Skipper a shot, too, with the happier feeling that it would protect him against the infection.

'One thing more, Jack,' I added. 'This disease also affects humans, so please take all hygienic precautions when handling Jingo. All right ?'

He nodded and lifted the bull terrier from the table. The big dog, as most of my patients do, tried to hurry away from the disturbing white-coat-and-antiseptic atmosphere of the surgery. As he trotted along the passage his master turned to me eagerly.

'Look at that! He doesn't seem too bad, does he ?'

I didn't say anything. I hoped with all my heart that he was right, but I was fighting off the conviction that this nice animal was doomed. At any rate I would soon know.

I knew, in fact, next day. Jack Sanders was on the phone before nine o'clock in the morning.

'Jing's not so good,' he said, but the tremor in his voice belied the lightness of his words.

'Oh.' I experienced the familiar drooping of the spirits. 'What is he doing?'

'Nothing, I'm afraid. Won't eat a thing ... lying around ... just lifeless. And every now and then he vomits.'

It was what I expected, but I still felt like kicking the desk by my side. 'Very well, I'll be right round.'

There were no tail wags from Jing today. He was crouched before the fire, gazing listlessly into the coals. The yellow in his eyes had deepened to a rich orange and his temperature still soared. I repeated the serum injection, but the big dog did not heed the entry of the needle. Before I left I ran my hand over the smooth white body and Skipper as ever kept burrowing in on his friend, but Jingo's thoughts were elsewhere, sunk in his inner misery.

I visited him daily and on the fourth day I found him stretched almost comatose on his side. The conjunctiva, sclera, and the mucous membranes of the mouth were a dirty chocolate colour.

'Is he suffering?' Jack Sanders asked.

I hesitated for a moment. 'I honestly don't think he's in pain. Sickness, nausea, yes, but I'd say that's all.'

'Well, I'd like to keep on trying,' he said. 'I don't want to put him down even though you think it's hopeless. You do ... don't you?'

I made a non-committal gesture. I was watching Skipper who seemed bewildered. He had given up his worrying tactics and was sniffing round his friend in a puzzled manner. Only once did he pull very gently at the unresponsive ear.

I went through the motions with a feeling of helplessness and left with the unpleasant intuition that I would never see Jingo alive again.

And even though I was waiting for it, Jack Sanders' phone call next morning was a bad start to the day.

'Jing died during the night, Mr Herriot. I thought I'd better let you know. You said you were coming back this morning.' He was trying to be matter-of-fact.

'I'm sorry, Jack,' I said. 'I did rather expect . . .'

'Yes, I know. And thank you for what you did.'

It made it worse when people were nice at these times. The Sanders were a childless couple and devoted to their animals. I knew how he was feeling.

I stood there with the receiver in my hand. 'Anyway, Jack, you've still got Skipper.' It sounded a bit lame, but it did help to have the comfort of one remaining dog, even though he was old.

'That's right,' he replied. 'We're very thankful for Skipper.'

I went on with my work. Patients died sometimes and once it was over it was almost a relief, especially when I knew in Jingo's case that the end was inevitable.

But this thing wasn't over. Less than a week later Jack Sanders was on the phone again.

'It's Skipper,' he said. 'He seems to be going the same way as Jing.'

A cold hand took hold of my stomach and twisted it.

'But . . . but . . . he can't be! I gave him the protective injection!'

'Well, I don't know, but he's hanging around miserably and hardly eats a thing. He seems to be going down fast.'

I ran out and jumped into my car. And as I drove to the edge of the town where the Sanders lived my heart thudded and panicky thoughts jostled around in my mind. How could he have got the infection? I had little faith in the serum as a cure but as a prevention I felt it was safe. I had even given him a second shot to make sure. The idea of these people losing both their dogs was bad enough but I couldn't bear the thought that the second one might be my fault.

The little corgi trailed unhappily across the carpet when he saw me and I lifted him quickly on to the kitchen table. I almost snatched at his eyelids in my anxiety but there was no sign of jaundice in the sclera nor in the mucous membranes of the mouth. The temperature was dead normal and I felt a wave of relief.

'He hasn't got leptospirosis, anyway,' I said.

Mrs Sanders clasped her hands. 'Oh, thank God for that. We were sure it was the same thing. He looks so awful.'

I examined the little animal meticulously and when I finished I put my stethoscope in my pocket. 'Well, I can't find much wrong here. He's got a bit of a heart murmur but you've known that for some time. He's old, after all.'

'Do you think he could be fretting for Jing?' Jack Sanders asked.

'Yes, I do. They were such friends. He must feel lost.'

'But he'll get over that, won't he?'

'Oh, of course he will. I'll leave some mild sedative tablets for him and I'm sure they'll help.'

I met Jack a few days later in the market place.

'How is Skipper?' I asked.

He blew out his cheeks. 'About the same. Maybe a bit worse. The trouble is he eats practically nothing – he's getting very thin.'

I didn't see what else I could do but on the following day I looked in at the Sanders' as I was passing.

I was shocked at the little corgi's appearance. Despite his age he had been so cocky and full of bounce, and when Jing was alive he had been indisputably the boss dog. But now he was utterly deflated. He looked at me with lack-lustre eyes as I came in, then crept stiffly to his basket where he curled himself as though wishing to shut out the world.

I examined him again. The heart murmur seemed a little more pronounced but there was nothing else except that he looked old and decrepit and done.

'You know, I'm beginning to wonder if he really is fretting.' I said. 'It could be just his age catching up on him. After all, he'll be twelve in the spring, won't he?'

Mrs Sanders nodded. 'That's right. Then you think . . . this could be the end?'

'It's possible.' I knew what she was thinking. A couple of weeks ago two healthy dogs rolling around and playing in this house and now there could soon be none.

'But isn't there anything else you can do?'

'Well, I can give him a course of digitalis for his heart. And perhaps you would bring in a sample of his urine. I want to see how his kidneys are functioning.'

I tested the urine. There was a little albumen, but no more than you would expect in a dog of his age. I ruled out nephritis as a cause.

As the days passed I tried other things; vitamins, iron tonics, organo-phosphates, but the little animal declined steadily. It was about a month after Jing's death that I called to the house again.

Skipper was in his basket and when I called to him he slowly raised his head. His face was pinched and fleshless and the filmed eyes regarded me without recognition.

'Come on, lad,' I said encouragingly. 'Let's see you get out of there.'

Jack Sanders shook his head. 'It's no good, Mr Herriot. He never leaves his basket now and when we lift him out he's almost too weak to walk. Another thing . . . he makes a mess down here in the kitchen during the night. That's something he's never done.'

It was like the tolling of a sad bell. Everything he said pointed to a dog in the last stages of senility. I tried to pick my words.

'I'm sorry, Jack, but it all sounds as if the old chap has come to the end of the road. I don't think fretting could possibly cause all this.'

He didn't speak for a moment. He looked at his wife then down at the forlorn little creature. 'Well, of course, this has been in the back of our minds. But we've kept hoping he would start to eat. What . . . what do you suggest?'

I could not bring myself to say the fateful words. 'It seems to me that we can't stand by and let him suffer. He's just a little skeleton and I can't think he's getting any pleasure out of his life now.'

'I see,' he said. 'And I agree. He lies there all day – he has no interest in anything.' He paused and looked at his wife again. 'I tell you what, Mr Herriot. Let us think it over till tomorrow. But you do think there's no hope?'

'Yes, Jack, I do. Old dogs often go this way at the end. Skipper has just cracked up . . . he's finished, I'm afraid.'

He drew a long breath. 'Right, if you don't hear from me by eight o'clock tomorrow morning, please come and put him to sleep.'

I had small hope of the call coming and it didn't. In those early days of our marriage Helen worked as a secretary for one of the local millers. We often started our day together by descending the long flights of stairs from our bed-sitter and I would see her out of the front door before getting ready for my round.

This morning she gave me her usual kiss before going out into the street but then she looked at me searchingly. 'You've been quiet all through breakfast, Jim. What's the matter?'

'It's nothing, really. Just part of the job,' I said. But when she kept her steady gaze on me I told her quickly about the Sanders.

She touched my arm. 'It's such a shame, Jim, but you can't let your sad cases depress you. You'd never survive.'

'Aagh, I know that. But I'm a softy, that's my trouble. Sometimes I think I should never have been a vet.'

'You're wrong there,' she said. 'I couldn't imagine you as anything else. You'll do what you have to do, and you'll do it the right way.' She kissed me again, turned and ran down the steps.

It was mid-morning before I drew up outside the Sanders' home. I opened the car boot and took out the syringe and the bottle of concentrated anaesthetic which would give the old dog a peaceful and painless end.

The first thing I saw when I went into the kitchen was a fat white puppy waddling across the floor.

I looked down in astonishment. 'What's this . . . ?'

Mrs Sanders gave me a strained smile, 'Jack and I had a talk yesterday. We couldn't bear the idea of not having a dog at all, so we went round to Mrs Palmer who bred Jing and found she had a litter for sale. It seemed like fate. We've called him Jingo, too.'

'What a splendid idea!' I lifted the pup which squirmed in my hand, grunted in an obese manner and tried to lick my face. This, I felt, would make my unpleasant task easier. 'I think you've been very sensible.'

I lifted the bottle of anaesthetic unobtrusively from my pocket and went over to the basket in the corner. Skipper was still curled in the unheeding ball of yesterday and the comforting thought came to me that all I was going to do was push him a little further along the journey he had already begun.

I pierced the rubber diaphragm on the bottle with my needle and was about to withdraw the barbiturate when I saw that Skipper had raised his head. Chin resting on the edge of the basket, he seemed to be watching the pup. Wearily his eyes followed the tiny creature as it made its way to a dish of milk and began to lap busily. And there was something in his intent expression which had not been there for a long time.

I stood very still as the corgi made a couple of attempts then heaved himself to a standing position. He almost fell out of the basket and staggered on shaking legs across the floor. When he came alongside the pup he remained there, swaying, for some time, a gaunt caricature of his former self, but as I watched in disbelief, he reached forward and seized the little white ear in his mouth.

Stoicism is not a characteristic of pups and Jingo the Second yelped shrilly as the teeth squeezed. Skipper, undeterred, continued to gnaw with rapt concentration.

I dropped bottle and syringe back in my pocket. 'Bring him some food,' I said quietly.

Mrs Sanders hurried to the pantry and came back with a few pieces of meat on a saucer. Skipper continued his ear-nibbling for a few moments then sniffed the pup unhurriedly from end to end before turning to the saucer. He hardly had the strength to chew but he lifted a portion of meat and his jaws moved slowly.

'Good heavens!' Jack Sanders burst out. 'That's the first thing he's eaten for days!'

His wife seized my arm. 'What's happened, Mr Herriot? We only got the puppy because we couldn't have a house without a dog.'

'Well, it looks to me as though you've got two again.' I went over to the door and smiled back at the two people watching fascinated as the corgi swallowed then started determinedly on another piece of meat. 'Good morning, I'm going now.'

About eight months later, Jack Sanders came into the surgery and put Jingo Two on the table. He was growing into a fine animal with the wide chest and powerful legs of the breed. His good-natured face and whipping tail reminded me strongly of his predecessor.

'He's got a bit of eczema between his pads,' Jack said, then he bent and lifted Skipper up.

At that moment I had no eyes for my patient. All my attention was on the corgi, plump and bright-eyed, nibbling at the big dog's hind limbs with all his old bounce and vigour.

'Just look at that!' I murmured. 'It's like turning the clock back.'

Jack Sanders laughed. 'Yes, isn't it. They're tremendous friends – just like before.'

'Come here, Skipper.' I grabbed the little corgi and looked him over. When I had finished I held him for a moment as he tried to wiggle his way back to his friend. 'Do you know, I honestly think he'll go on for years yet.'

'Really?' Jack Sanders looked at me with a mischievous light in his eyes. 'But I seem to remember you saying quite a long time ago that his days were over – he was finished.'

I held up a hand, 'I know, I know. But sometimes it's lovely to be wrong.'

5

'That young Herriot's a bloody thick-'ead.'

It wasn't the sort of statement to raise one's morale and for a moment the good ale turned to vinegar in my mouth. I was having a quiet pint all alone in the 'snug' of the Crown and Anchor on my way home from an evening colic case, and the words came clearly through the hatch from the public bar.

I suppose it was the fact that I had come to the conclusion that my flying instructor, FO Woodham, considered me to be a person of low intelligence that brought the incident back to my mind.

I shifted my position slightly so that I could see into the brightly lit room. The speaker was Seth Pilling, a casual labourer and a well-known character in Darrowby. He was designated a labourer, but in truth he didn't labour unduly and his burly frame and red meaty face was a common sight around the Labour Exchange where he signed for his unemployment pay.

'Aye, 'e's got no idea. Knaws nowt about dogs.' The big man tipped about half a pint over his throat in one swallow.

'He's not a bad hand wi' cows,' another voice broke in.

'Aye, maybe, but I'm not talkin' about bloody awd cows,' Seth retorted witheringly. 'I'm talkin' about dogs. Ye need skill to doctor dogs.'

A third man spoke up. 'Well, 'e's a vitnery, isn't he ?'

'Aye, a knaw he is, but there's all kind o' vitneries and this 'un's a dead loss. Ah could tell ye some tales about this feller.'

They say an eavesdropper never hears anything good about himself, and I knew the sensible thing would be to get out of there immediately rather than hear this man vilifying me in a crowded bar. But of course I didn't get out. I stayed, morbidly fascinated, listening with every nerve and fibre.

'What sort o' tales, Seth ?' The company was as interested as I was.

'Well,' he replied. 'There's many a time folks 'ave brought dogs to me that he's made a mess of.'

'Tha knaws all about dogs, doesn't tha, Seth ?'

It was perhaps wishful thinking that made me imagine a touch of sarcasm in the last remark, but if it were so it was lost on Mr Pilling. His big, stupid face creased into a self-satisfied smirk.

'Ah'll tell ye there's not a lot ah don't know about 'em. I've been among 'em all me life and I've studied t'job, too.' He slurped down more beer. 'I've got a houseful o' books and read 'em all. Ah ken everythin' about them diseases and the remedies.'

Another of the men in the bar spoke. 'Have you ever been beat wi' a dog job, Seth ?'

There was a pause. 'Well, ah'm not goin' to say I never 'ave,' he said judicially. 'It's very rare I'm beat, but if I am I don't go to Herriot.' He shook his head. 'Nay, nay, ah slip through to Brawton and consult wi' Dennaby Broome. He's a big friend o' mine.'

In the quiet of the snug I sipped at my glass. Dennaby Broome was one of the many 'quacks' who flourished in those days. He had started in the building trade – as a plasterer to be exact – and had gravitated mysteriously and without formal training into the field of veterinary science where he now made a comfortable living.

I had nothing against him for that – we all have to live. In any case he rarely bothered me because Brawton was mainly outside

52

our practice orbit, but my colleagues around there used some unkind words about him. I had a private conviction that a lot of his success was due to his resounding name. To me, the very words 'Dennaby Broome' were profoundly imposing.

'Aye, that's what ah do,' Seth continued. 'Dennaby and me's big friends and we oft consult about dogs. Matter of fact ah took me own dog to 'im once – he looks well, eh ?'

I stood on tiptoe and peered into the bar. I could just see Seth's keeshound sitting at his feet. A handsome creature with a luxuriant glossy coat. The big man leaned over and patted the fox-like head. 'He's a vallible animal is that. Ah couldn't trust 'im to a feller like Herriot.'

'What's the matter wi' Herriot, any road ?' somebody asked.

'Well, ah'll tell tha.' Seth tapped his head. 'He hasn't got ower much up 'ere.'

I didn't want to hear any more. I put down my glass and stole out into the night.

After that experience I took more notice of Seth Pilling. He was often to be seen strolling round the town because, despite his vast store of knowledge on many subjects, he was frequently out of work. He wasn't an expert only on dogs – he pontificated in the Crown and Anchor on politics, gardening, cage birds, agriculture, the state of the economy, cricket, fishing and many other matters. There were few topics which his wide intellect did not effortlessly embrace, so that it was surprising that employers seemed to dispense with his services after a very brief period.

He usually took his dog with him on his strolls, and the attractive animal began to appear to me as a symbol of my shortcomings. Instinctively I kept out of his way but one morning I came right up against him.

It was at the little shelter in the market place and a group of people were waiting for the Brawton bus. Among them was Seth Pilling and the keeshound, and as I passed within a few feet of them on my way to the post office I stopped involuntarily and stared. The dog was almost unrecognizable.

The dense, off-standing ash-grey coat I knew so well had become sparse and lustreless. The thick ruff, so characteristic of the breed, had shrunk to nothing.

'You're lookin' at me dog?' Mr Pilling tightened the lead and pulled the little animal towards him protectively as though he feared I might put my contaminated hand on him.

'Yes . . . I'm sorry, but I couldn't help noticing. He has a skin condition . . . ?'

The big man looked down his nose at me. 'Aye, 'e has, a bit. I'm just takin' him through to Brawton to see Dennaby Broome.'

'I see.'

'Yes, ah thought ah'd better take 'im to somebody as knows summat about dogs.' He smirked as he looked around at the people in the shelter who were listening with interest. 'He's a vallible dog is that.'

'I'm sure he is,' I said.

He raised his voice further. 'Mind you, ah've been givin' him some of me own treatment.' He didn't have to tell me. There was a strong smell of tar, and the dog's hair was streaked with some oily substance. 'But it's maybe better to make sure. We're lucky to 'ave a man like Dennaby Broome to turn to.'

'Quite.'

He looked around his audience appreciatively. 'Especially with a vallible dog like this. You can't 'ave any Tom Dick or Harry muckin' around with 'im.'

'Well,' I said. 'I hope you get him put right.'

'Oh, ah will.' The big man was enjoying the interlude, and he laughed. 'Don't *you* worry about *that*.'

This little session did not enliven my day, but it gave me more reason to watch out for Mr Pilling. For the next two weeks I observed his movements with the deepest interest because his dog was losing its hair at an alarming rate. Not only that, but the animal's whole demeanour had changed and instead of tripping along in his old sprightly way he dragged one foot after another as though he were on the point of death.

Towards the end of the period I was horrified to see the big man with something like a shorn ewe on the end of the lead. It was all that was left of the beautiful keeshound, but as I started to walk towards him his master spotted me and hurried off in the opposite direction, dragging the unfortunate animal behind him.

I did, however, succeed in having a look at the dog a few days afterwards. He was in the waiting room at Skeldale House, and this time he was accompanied by his mistress instead of his master.

Mrs Pilling was sitting very upright, and when I asked her to come through to the consulting room she jumped to her feet, marched past me and stumped quickly along the passage in front of me.

She was quite small, but broad hipped and stocky, and she always walked rapidly, her head nodding forward aggressively at each step, her jaw thrust out. She never smiled.

I had heard it said that Seth Pilling was a big talker outside, but under his own roof he was scared to death of his little wife. And as the tight-mouthed fiery-eyed face turned to me I could believe it.

She bent, pushed powerful arms under the keeshound and hoisted him on to the table.

'Just look at me dog, Mr Herriot!' She rapped out.

I looked. 'Good heavens!' I gasped.

The little animal was almost completely bald. His skin was dry, scaly and wrinkled, and his head hung down as though he were under sedation.

'Aye, you're surprised, aren't you?' she barked. 'And no wonder. He's in a terrible state, isn't he?'

'I'm afraid so. I wouldn't have known him.'

'No, nobody would. Ah think the world 'o this dog and just look at 'im!' She paused and snorted a few times. 'And I know who's responsible, don't you?'

'Well...'

'Oh, you do. It's that husband o' mine.' She paused and glared at me, breathing rapidly. 'What d'you think of my husband, Mr Herriot?'

'I really don't know him very well. I...'

'Well, ah know 'im and he's a gawp. He's a great gawp. Knows everything and knows nowt. He's played around wi' me good dog till he's ruined 'im.'

I didn't say anything. I was studying the keeshound. It was the first time I had been able to observe him closely and I was certain I knew the cause of the trouble.

Mrs Pilling stuck her jaw out further and continued.

'First me husband said it was eczema. Is it?'

'No.'

'Then 'e said it was mange. Is it?'

'No.'

'D'you know what it is?'

'Yes.'

'Well, will you tell me please?'

'It's myxoedema.'

'Myx...?'

'Wait a minute,' I said. 'I'll just make absolutely sure.' I reached for my stethoscope and put it on the dog's chest. And the bradycardia was there as I expected, the slow, slow heartbeat of hypothyroidism. 'Yes, that's it. Not a shadow of a doubt about it.'

'What did you call it?'

'Myxoedema. It's a thyroid deficiency – there's a gland in his neck which isn't doing its job properly.'

'And that makes 'is hair fall out?'

'Oh yes. And it also causes this typical scaliness and wrinkling of the skin.'

'Aye, but he's half asleep all t'time. How about that?'

'Another classical symptom. Dogs with this condition become very lethargic – lose all their energy.'

She reached out and touched the dog's skin, bare and leathery where once the coat had grown in bushy glory. 'And can you cure it?'

'Yes.'

'Now Mr Herriot, don't take this the wrong way, but could you be mistaken? Are ye positive it's this myxi-whatever-it-is?'

'Of course I am. It's a straightforward case.'

'Straightforward to you, maybe.' She flushed and appeared to be grinding her teeth. 'But not straightforward to that clever husband o' mine. The great lubbert! When ah think what he's put me good dog through – ah could kill 'im.'

'Well, I suppose he thought he was acting for the best, Mrs Pilling.'

'Ah don't care what he thought, he's made this poor dog suffer, the big fool. Wait till ah get hold of 'im.'

I gave her a supply of tablets. 'These are thyroid extract, and I want you to give him one night and morning.' I also handed her a bottle of potassium iodide which I had found helpful in these cases.

She looked at me doubtfully. 'But surely he'll want summat rubbed on 'is skin.'

'No,' I replied. 'Applications to the skin do no good at all.'

'Then you mean.' She turned a dark purple colour and began snorting again. 'You mean all them bottles o' filthy stuff me husband put on 'im were a waste o' time?'

'Afraid so.'

'Oh, ah'll murder 'im!' she burst out. 'Mucky, oily rubbish, it was. And that fancy feller in Brawton sent some 'orrible lotion – yeller it was, and stank the place out. Ruined me carpets and good chair covers an' all!'

Sulphur, whale oil and creosote, I thought. Splendid old-fashioned ingredients, but quite useless in this case and definitely antisocial.

Mrs Pilling heaved the keeshound to the floor and strode along the passage, head down, powerful shoulders hunched. I could hear her muttering to herself as she went.

'By gaw, just wait till ah get home. Ah'll sort 'im, by gaw ah will!'

I was naturally interested in the progress of my patient, and when I failed to see him around for the next fortnight I could only conclude that Seth Pilling was keeping out of my way. Indeed there was one occasion when I thought I saw him and the dog disappearing down an alley, but I couldn't be sure.

When I did see them both it was by accident. I was driving round the corner into the market place and I came upon a man and dog coming away from one of the stalls on the cobbles.

And as I peered through the window I caught my breath. Even in that short space of time the animal's skin was covered with a healthy down of new hair, and he was stepping out with something like his old vitality.

His master swung round as I slowed down. He gave me a single hunted look then tugged on the lead and scuttled away.

I could only imagine the turmoil in his mind, the conflict of emotions. No doubt he wanted to see his dog recover, but not this way. And as it turned out, the dice were loaded against the poor man because this was an unbelievably rapid recovery. I have seen some spectacular cures in myxoedema, but none so dramatic as that keeshound.

Mr Pilling's sufferings were communicated to me in various ways. For instance I heard he had changed his pub and now went to the Red Bear of an evening. In a little place like Darrowby, news fairly crackles around and I had a good idea that the farm men in the Crown and Anchor would have had a bit of quiet Yorkshire sport with the expert.

But his main martyrdom was at home. It was about six weeks after I had finished treating the dog that Mrs Pilling brought him to the surgery.

As before, she lifted him easily on to the table and looked at me, her face as always grim and unsmiling.

'Mr Herriot,' she said. 'Ah've just come to say thank ye, and ah thought you'd be interested to see me dog now.'

'I am indeed, Mrs Pilling. It's nice of you to come.' I gazed wonderingly at the thick coat, bushy, shining and new, and at the sparkling eyes and alert expression. 'I think you can say he's about back to normal.'

She nodded. 'That's what I thought and ah'm grateful to ye for what you've done.'

I walked with her to the front door and as she led her dog on to the street she turned her tough little face to me again. As the stern eyes met mine she looked very menacing.

'There's one thing,' she said. 'Ah'll never forgive that man o' mine for what he did to me dog. By gum, I've given 'im some stick, the great goof! He'll never hear the last of it from me.'

As she made off down the street, the little animal trotting briskly by her side, I brimmed with pleasant emotions. It is always warming to see a case recover so well, but in this instance there was an additional bonus.

For a long time little Mrs Pilling was going to give her husband pure hell.

6

'Today,' said FO Woodham, 'we're going to try a few new things. Spinning, sideslipping and how to come out of a stall.' His voice was gentle, and before he pulled on his helmet he turned his dark, fine-featured face towards me and smiled. Walking over the grass I thought what a likeable chap he was. I could have made a friend of him.

But he was always like that on the ground. He was altogether different in the air.

Yet I could never understand it. Flying was no trouble at all, and as we spun and dropped and soared about the summer sky his instructions appeared simple and easy to carry out. But the rot, as always, began to set in very soon.

'Didn't I tell you opposite rudder and stick to sideslip?' he bawled over the intercom.

'Yes, sir,' was all I replied, instead of the more appropriate, 'That's just what I'm doing, you stupid bugger!' which I might have used in civil life.

The goggled eyes bulged in the mirror. 'Well, why the bloody hell aren't you doing it?' His voice rose to a wild shriek.

'Sorry, sir.'

'Well, take her up. We'll try again. And for God's sake keep your wits about you!'

It was the same with the spins and stalls. I hadn't the slightest difficulty in pulling out of them but at times I thought my instructor was going out of his mind.

Berserk cries rang in my ears. 'Full opposite rudder and centralize the stick! Centralize it! Can't you hear me? Oh God, God!'

And of course the panic gradually crept in and I began to crack. One moment I could see a railway station in front of me whirling around in crazy circles, then there was nothing but the empty heavens and within seconds fields and trees would start to rush at me. Everything kept changing bewilderingly except the enraged eyes in the mirror and the exasperated yells.

'Centralize it, you bloody fool! Keep your eye on that cloud!

Watch your artificial horizon! Don't you know what the altimeter's for? I told you to keep at one thousand feet but it's like talking to a bloody wall!'

After a while a kind of numbness took over and the words rang meaninglessly in my head, one sentence seeming to contradict another. Desperately I tried to sort out the volleys of advice, but the whole thing began to slip from my grasp.

I had felt like this somewhere before. There was a familiar ring about this jumble in my brain. Then it came back to me. It was like being back at the Birtwhistles.

The trouble with the Birtwhistles was that they all spoke at once. Mr Birtwhistle invariably discussed his livestock, his wife concentrated on family matters and Len, their massive eighteen-year-old son, talked of nothing but football.

I was examining Nellie, the big white cow that always stood opposite the doorway in the grey stone byre. She had been lame for over a week and I didn't like the look of her.

'Lift her foot, will you, Len,' I said. It was wonderful to have a muscular giant to hoist the hind limb instead of going through the tedious business of hauling it up with a rope over a beam.

With the cloven hoof cradled in the great hands I could see that my fears were realized. The space between the cleats was clear but there was a significant swelling around the interphalangeal joint.

I looked up from my stooping position. 'Can you see that, Mr Birtwhistle? The infection is spreading upwards.'

'Aye . . . aye . . .' The farmer thrust a finger against the tumefied area and Nellie flinched. 'It's goin' up her leg on that side right enough. Ah thought it was nowt but a bit o' foul and I've been puttin' . . .'

'By gaw,' Len interjected. 'The lads 'ad a good win against Hellerby on Saturday. Johnnie Nudd got another couple o' goals and . . .'

' . . . puttin' that caustic lotion between 'er cleats.' Mr Birtwhistle didn't appear to have heard his son, but it was always like that. 'Done it regular night and mornin'. And ah'll tell ye the best way to do it. Get a hen feather an' . . .'

' . . . ah wouldn't be surprised if 'e scores a few more this

Saturday,' continued Len unheedingly. 'He's a right bobby dazzler when 'e . . .'

'. . . ye just dip it in t'lotion and push the feather in between t'cleats. It works like a . . .'

'. . . gets that ball on 'is right foot. He just whacks 'em in . . .'

I raised a hand. 'Wait a minute. You must realize this cow hasn't got foul. She has suppurative arthritis in this little joint just at the coronet here. I don't want to use a lot of big words but she has pus – matter – right inside the joint cavity, and it's a very nasty thing.'

Mr Birtwhistle nodded slowly. 'Sort of a abscess, you mean? Well, maybe it ud be best to lance it. Once you let t'matter out it would . . .'

'. . . just like a rocket,' went on Len. 'Ah'll tell ye, Johnnie could get a trial for Darlington one o' these days and then . . .'

I always think it is polite to look at a person when they are talking to you, but it is difficult when they are both talking at once, especially when one of them is bent double and the other standing behind you.

'Thank you, Len,' I said. 'You can put her foot down now.' I straightened up and directed my gaze somewhere between them. 'The trouble with this condition is that you can't just stick a knife into it and relieve it. Very often the smooth surfaces of the joint are eaten away and it's terribly painful.'

Nellie would agree with me. It was the outside cleat which was affected and she was standing with her leg splayed sideways in an attempt to take the weight on the healthy inner digit.

The farmer asked the inevitable question. 'Well, what are we goin' to do?'

I had an uncomfortable conviction that it wasn't going to make much difference what we did, but I had to make an effort.

'We'll give her a course of sulphanilamide powders and I also want you to put a poultice on that foot three times daily.'

'Poultice?' The farmer brightened. 'Ah've been doin' that. Ah've been . . .'

'If Darlington signed Johnnie Nudd I reckon . . .'

'Hold on, Len,' I said. 'What poultice have you been using, Mr Birtwhistle?'

'Cow shit,' the farmer replied confidently. 'Ye can't beat a good cow shit poultice to bring t'bad out. Ah've used it for them bad cases o' . . .'

'. . . ah'd have to go through to Darlington now and then instead of watchin' the Kestrels,' Len broke in. 'Ah'd have to see how Johnnie was gettin' on wi' them professionals because . . .'

I managed a twisted smile. I like football myself and I found it touching that Len ignored the great panorama of league football to concentrate on a village team who played in front of about twenty spectators. 'Yes, yes, Len, I quite understand how you feel.' Then I turned to his father. 'I was thinking of a rather different type of poultice, Mr Birtwhistle.'

The farmer's face lengthened and the corners of his mouth drooped. 'Well, ah've never found owt better than cow shit and ah've been among stock all me life.'

I clenched my teeth. This earthy medicament was highly regarded among the Dales farmers of the thirties and the damnable thing was that it often achieved its objective. There was no doubt that a sackful of bovine faeces applied to an inflamed area set up a tremendous heat and counter-irritation. In those days I had to go along with many of the ancient cures and keep my tongue between my teeth but I never prescribed cow shit and I wasn't going to start now.

'Maybe so,' I said firmly, 'but what I was thinking of was kaolin. You could call down at the surgery for some. You just heat the tin in a pan of hot water and apply the poultice to the foot. It keeps its heat for several hours.'

Mr Birtwhistle showed no great enthusiasm so I tried again.

'Or you could use bran. I see you've got a sack over there.'

He cheered up a little. 'Aye . . . that's right.'

'Okay, put on some hot bran three times a day and give her the powders and I'll see her again in a few days.' I knew the farmer would do as I said, because he was a conscientious stockman, but I had seen cases like this before and I wasn't happy. Nothing seems to pull a good cow down quicker than a painful foot. Big fat animals could be reduced to skeletons within weeks because of the agony of septic arthritis. I could only hope.

'Very good, Mr Herriot,' Mr Birtwhistle said. 'And now come into the house. T'missus has a cup o' tea ready for you.'

I seldom refuse such an invitation but as I entered the kitchen I knew this was where the going got really tough.

'Now then, Mr Herriot,' the farmer's wife said, beaming as she handed me a steaming mug. 'I was talkin' to your good lady in the market place yesterday, and she said . . .'

'And ye think them powders o' yours might do the trick?' Her husband looked at me seriously. 'I 'ope so, because Nellie's a right good milker. Ah reckon last lactation she gave . . .'

'Kestrels is drawn agin Dibham in t'Hulton cup.' Len chimed in. 'It'll be some game. Last time . . .'

Mrs Birtwhistle continued without drawing breath. '. . . you were nicely settled in at top of Skeldale House. It must be right pleasant up there with the lovely view and . . .'

'. . . five gallons when she fust calved and she kept it up for . . .'

'. . . they nearly kicked us off t'pitch, but by gaw ah'll tell ye, we'll . . .'

'. . . you can see right over Darrowby. But it wouldn't do for a fat body like me. I was sayin' to your missus that you 'ave to be young and slim to live up there. All them stairs and . . .'

I took a long draught from my cup. It gave me a chance to focus my eyes and attention on just one thing as the conversation crackled unceasingly around me. I invariably found it wearing trying to listen to all three Birtwhistles in full cry and of course it was impossible to look at them all simultaneously and adjust my expression to their different remarks.

The thing that amazed me was that none of them ever became angry at the others butting in. Nobody ever said, 'I'm speaking, do you mind?' or 'Don't interrupt!' or 'For Pete's sake, shut up!' They lived together in perfect harmony with all of them talking at once and none paying the slightest heed to what the other was saying.

When I saw the cow during the following week she was worse. Mr Birtwhistle had followed my instructions faithfully but Nellie could scarcely hobble as he brought her in from the field.

Len was there to lift the foot and I gloomily surveyed the increased swelling. It ran right round the coronet from the heel to the interdigital cleft in front, and the slightest touch from my finger caused the big cow to jerk her leg in pain.

I didn't say much, because I knew what was in store for Nellie and I knew too, that Mr Birtwhistle wasn't going to like it when I told him.

When I visited again at the end of the week I had only to look at the farmer's face to realize that everything had turned out as I feared. For once he was on his own and he led me silently to the byre.

Nellie was on three legs now, not daring even to bring the infected foot into momentary contact with the cobbled flooring. And worse, she was in an advanced state of emaciation, the sleek healthy animal of two weeks ago reduced to little more than bone and hide.

'I doubt she's 'ad it,' Mr Birtwhistle muttered.

Cow's hind feet are difficult to lift, but today I didn't need any help because Nellie had stopped caring. I examined the swollen digit. It was now vast – a great ugly club of tissue with a trickle of pus discharging down the wall.

'I see it's bust there.' The farmer poked a finger at the ragged opening. 'But it hasn't given 'er no relief.'

'Well, I wouldn't expect it to,' I said. 'Remember I told you the trouble is all inside the joint.'

'Well, these things 'appen,' he replied. 'Ah might as well telephone for Mallock. She's hardly givin' a drop o' milk, poor awd lass, she's nawt but a screw now.'

I always had to wait for the threat of the knacker man's humane killer before I said what I had to say now. Right from the start this had been a case for surgery, but it would have been a waste of time to suggest it at the beginning. Amputation of the bovine digit has always filled farmers with horror and even now I knew I would have trouble convincing Mr Birtwhistle.

'There's no need to slaughter her,' I said. 'There's another way of curing this.'

'Another way ? We've tried 'ard enough, surely.'

I bent and lifted the foot again. 'Look at this.' I seized the inner cleat and moved it freely around. 'This side is perfectly healthy. There's nothing wrong with it. It would bear Nellie's full weight.'

'Aye, but . . . how about t'other 'orrible thing ?'

'I could remove it.'

'You mean . . . cut it off?'

'Yes.'

He shook his head vigorously 'Nay, nay, I'm not havin' that. She's suffered enough. Far better send for Jeff Mallock and get the job over.'

Here it was again. Farmers are anything but shrinking violets, but there was something about this business which appalled them.

'But Mr Birtwhistle,' I said. 'Don't you see – the pain is immediately relieved. The pressure is off and all the weight rests on the good side.'

'Ah said no, Mr Herriot, and ah mean no. You've done your best and I thank ye, but I'm not havin' her foot cut off and that's all about it.' He turned and began to walk away.

I looked after him helplessly. One thing I hate to do is talk a man into an operation on one of his beasts for the simple reason that if anything goes wrong I get the blame. But, as I was just about certain that an hour's work could restore this good cow to her former state, I couldn't let it go at this.

I trotted from the byre. The farmer was already halfway across the yard on his way to the phone.

I panted up to him as he reached the farmhouse door. 'Mr Birtwhistle, listen to me for a minute. I never said anything about cutting off her foot. Just one cleat.'

'Well that's half a foot, isn't it?' he looked down at his boots. 'And it's ower much for me.'

'But she wouldn't know a thing,' I pleaded. 'She'd be under a general anaesthetic. And I'm nearly sure it would be a success.'

'Mr Herriot, I just don't fancy it. I don't like t'idea. And even if it did work it would be like havin' a crippled cow walkin' about.'

'Not at all. She would grow a little stump of horn there and I'd like to bet you'd never notice a thing.'

He gave me a long sideways look and I could see he was weakening.

'Mr Birtwhistle,' I said, pressing home the attack. 'Within a month Nellie could be a fat cow again, giving five gallons of milk a day.'

This was silly talk, not to be recommended to any veterinary surgeon, but I was seized by a kind of madness. I couldn't bear the thought of that cow being cut up for dog food when I was convinced I could put it right. And there was another thing; I was already savouring the pleasure, childish perhaps, of instantly relieving an animal's pain, of bringing off a spectacular cure. There aren't many operations in the field of bovine surgery where you can do this but digit amputation is one of them.

Something of my fervour must have been communicated to the farmer because he looked at me steadily for a few moments then shrugged.

'When do you want to do it ?' he asked.

'Tomorrow.'

'Right. Will you need a lot o' fellers to help ?'

'No, just you and Len. I'll see you at ten o'clock.'

Next day the sun was warm on my back as I laid out my equipment on a small field near the house. It was a typical setting for many large animal operations I have carried out over the years; the sweet stretch of green, the grey stone buildings and the peaceful bulk of the fells rising calm and unheeding into the white scattering clouds.

It took a long time for them to lead Nellie out, though she didn't have far to go, and as the bony scarecrow hopped painfully towards me, dangling her useless limb, the brave words of yesterday seemed foolhardy.

'All right,' I said. 'Stop there. That's a good spot.' On the grass, nearby, lay my tray with the saw, chloroform, bandages, cotton wool and iodoform. I had my long casting rope too, which we used to pull cattle down, but I had a feeling Nellie wouldn't need it.

I was right. I buckled on the muzzle, poured some chloroform on to the sponge and the big white cow sank almost thankfully on to the cool green herbage.

'Kestrels had a smashin' match on Wednesday night,' Len chuckled happily. 'Johnnie Nudd didn't score but Len Bottomley . . .'

'I 'ope we're doin' t'right thing,' muttered Mr Birtwhistle. 'The way she staggered out 'ere I'd say it was a waste of time to . . .'

'. . . cracked in a couple o' beauties.' Len's face lit up at the memory. 'Kestrels is lucky to 'ave two fellers like . . .'

'Get hold of that bad foot, Len!' I barked, playing them at their own game. 'And keep it steady on that block of wood. And you, Mr Birtwhistle, hold her head down. I don't suppose she'll move, but if she does we'll have to give her more chloroform.'

Cows are good subjects for chloroform anaesthesia but I don't like to keep them laid out too long in case of regurgitation of food. I was in a hurry.

I quickly tied a bandage above the hoof, pulling it tight to serve as a tourniquet, then I reached back to the tray for the saw. The books are full of sophisticated methods of digit amputation with much talk of curved incisions, reflections of skin to expose the region of the articulations, and the like. But I have whipped off hundreds of cleats with a few brisk strokes of the saw below the coronary band with complete success.

I took a long breath. 'Hold tight, Len,' And set to work.

For a few moments there was silence except for the rhythmic grating of metal on bone, then the offending digit was lying on the grass, leaving a flat stump from which a few capillary vessels spurted. Using curved scissors I speedily disarticulated the remains of the bone from the second phalanx and held it up.

'Look at that!' I cried. 'Almost eaten away.' I pointed to the necrotic tissue in and around the joint. 'And d'you see all that rubbish? No wonder she was in pain.' I did a bit of quick curetting, dusted the surface with iodoform, applied a thick pad of cotton wool and prepared to bandage.

And as I tore the paper from the white rolls I felt a stab of remorse. In my absorption I had been rather rude. I had never replied to Len's remark about his beloved team. Maybe I could pass the next few minutes with a little gentle banter.

'Hey, Len,' I said. 'When you're talking about the Kestrels you never mention the time Willerton beat them five nil. How is that?'

In reply the young man hurled himself unhesitatingly at me, butting me savagely on the forehead. The assault of the great coarse-haired head against my skin was like being attacked by a curly-polled bull, and the impact sent me flying backwards on to the grass. At first the inside of my cranium was illuminated

by a firework display but as consciousness slipped away my last
sensation was of astonishment and disbelief.

I loved football myself but never had I thought that Len's
devotion to the Kestrels would lead him to physical violence. He
had always seemed a most gentle and harmless boy.

I suppose I was out for only a few seconds but I fancy I might
have spent a good deal longer lying on the cool turf but for the
fact that something kept hammering out the message that I was
in the middle of a surgical procedure. I blinked and sat up.

Nellie was still sleeping peacefully against the green background
of hills. Mr Birtwhistle, hands on her neck, was regarding me
anxiously, and Len was lying unconscious face down across the
cow's body.

'Has he hurt tha, Mr Herriot ?'

'No . . . no . . . not really. What happened ?'

'I owt to have told ye. He can't stand the sight o' blood. Great
daft beggar.' The farmer directed an exasperated glare at his
slumbering son. 'But ah've never seen 'im go down as fast as that.
Pitched right into you, 'e did!'

I rolled the young man's inert form to one side and began
again. I bandaged slowly and carefully because of the danger of
post-operative haemorrhage. I finished with several layers of
zinc oxide plaster then turned to the farmer.

'You can take her muzzle off now, Mr Birtwhistle. The job's
done.'

I was starting to wash my instruments in the bucket when
Len sat up almost as suddenly as he had slumped down. He was
deathly pale but he looked at me with his usual friendly smile.

'What was that ye were sayin' about t'Kestrels, Mr Herriot ?'

'Nothing, Len,' I replied hastily. 'Nothing at all.'

After three days I returned and removed the original dressing
which was caked hard with blood and pus. I dusted the stump
with powder again and bandaged on a clean soft pad of cotton
wool.

'She'll feel a lot more comfortable now,' I said, and indeed
Nellie was already looking vastly happier. She was taking some
weight on the affected foot – rather gingerly, as though she

couldn't believe that terrible thing had gone from her life.

As she walked away I crossed my fingers. The only thing that can ruin these operations is if the infection spreads to the other side. The inevitable result then is immediate slaughter and terrible disappointment.

But it never happened to Nellie. When I took off the second dressing she was almost sound and I didn't see her again until about five weeks after the operation.

I had finished injecting one of Mr Birtwhistle's pigs when I asked casually, 'And how's Nellie?'

'Come and 'ave a look at her,' the farmer replied. 'She's just in that field at side of t'road.'

We walked together over the grass to where the white cow was standing among her companions, head down, munching busily. And she must have done a lot of that since I saw her because she was fat again.

'Get on, lass.' The farmer gently nudged her rump with his thumb and she ambled forward a few paces before setting to work on another patch of grass. There wasn't the slightest trace of lameness.

'Well, that's grand,' I said. 'And is she milking well, too?'

'Aye, back to five gallons.' He pulled a much dented tobacco tin from his pocket, unscrewed the lid and produced an ancient watch. 'It's ten o'clock, young man. Len'll have gone into t'house for his tea, and 'lowance. Will ye come in and have a cup?'

I squared my shoulders and followed him inside, and the barrage began immediately.

'Summat right funny happened on Saturday,' Len said with a roar of laughter. 'Walter Gimmett was refereein' and 'e gave two penalties agin t'Kestrels. So what did the lads do, they . . .'

'Eee, wasn't it sad about old Mr Brent?' Mrs Birtwhistle put her head on one side and looked at me piteously. 'We buried 'im on Saturday and . . .'

'You know, Mr Herriot,' her husband put in. 'Ah thought you were pullin' ma leg when you said Nellie would be givin' five gallons again. I never . . .'

'. . . dumped the beggar in a 'oss trough. He won't give no more penalties agin t'Kestrels. You should 'ave seen . . .'

'. . . it would 'ave been his ninetieth birthday today, poor old man. He was well liked in t'village and there was a big congregation. Parson said . . .'

'. . . expected owt like that. Ah thought she might maybe put on a bit of flesh so we could get 'er off for beef. Ah'm right grateful to . . .'

At that moment, fingers clenched tensely around my cup, I happened to catch sight of my reflection in a cracked mirror above the kitchen sink. It was a frightening experience because I was staring glassily into space with my features contorted almost out of recognition. There was something of an idiot smile as I acknowledged the humour of Walter in the horse trough, a touch of sorrow at Mr Brent's demise, and, I swear, a suggestion of gratification at the successful outcome of Nellie's operation. And since I was also trying to look in three directions at once, I had to give myself full marks for effort.

But as I say, I found it a little unnerving and excused myself soon afterwards. The men were still busy with Mrs Birtwhistle's apple pie and scones and the conversation was raging unabated when I left. The closure of the door behind me brought a sudden peace. The feeling of tranquillity stayed with me as I got into my car and drove out of the yard and on to the narrow country road. It persisted as I stopped the car after less than a hundred yards and wound down the window to have a look at my patient.

Nellie was lying down now. She had eaten her fill and was resting comfortably on her chest as she chewed her cud. To a doctor of farm animals there is nothing more reassuring than that slow lateral grinding. It means contentment and health. She gazed at me across the stone wall and the placid eyes in the white face added to the restfulness of the scene, accentuating the silence after the babel of voices in the farmhouse.

Nellie couldn't talk, but those calmly moving jaws told me all I wanted to know.

7

To me there are few things more appealing than a dog begging.
This one was tied to a lamp post outside a shop in Windsor. Its
eyes were fixed steadfastly on the shop doorway, willing its
owner to come out, and every now and then it sat up in mute
entreaty.

Flying had been suspended for an afternoon. It gave us all a
chance to relax and no doubt it eased the frayed nerves of our
instructors, but as I looked at that dog all the pressures of the
RAF fell away and I went back to Darrowby.

It was when Siegfried and I were making one of our market
day sorties that we noticed the little dog among the stalls.

When things were quiet in the surgery we often used to walk
together across the cobbles and have a word with the farmers
gathered round the doorway of the Drovers' Arms. Sometimes
we collected a few outstanding bills or drummed up a bit of work
for the forthcoming week – and if nothing like that happened we
still enjoyed the fresh air.

The thing that made us notice the dog was that he was sitting
up begging in front of the biscuit stall.

'Look at that little chap,' Siegfried said. 'I wonder where he's
sprung from.'

As he spoke, the stallholder threw a biscuit which the dog
devoured eagerly but when the man came round and stretched
out a hand the little animal trotted away.

He stopped, however, at another stall which sold produce:
eggs, cheese, butter, cakes and scones. Without hesitation he sat
up again in the begging position, rock steady, paws dangling,
head pointing expectantly.

I nudged Siegfried. 'There he goes again.'

My colleague nodded. 'Yes, he's an engaging little thing, isn't
he ? What breed would you call him ?'

'A cross, I'd say. He's like a little brown sheepdog, but there's
a touch of something else – maybe terrier.'

It wasn't long before he was munching a bun, and this time we
walked over to him. And as we drew near I spoke gently.

'Here, boy,' I said, squatting down a yard away. 'Come on, let's have a look at you.'

He faced me and for a moment two friendly brown eyes gazed at me from a singularly attractive little face. The fringed tail waved in response to my words but as I inched nearer he turned and ambled unhurriedly among the market day crowd till he was lost to sight. I didn't want to make a thing out of the encounter because I could never quite divine Siegfried's attitude to the small animals. He was eminently wrapped up in his horse work and often seemed amused at the way I rushed around after dogs and cats.

At that time, in fact, Siegfried was strongly opposed to the whole idea of keeping animals as pets. He was quite vociferous on the subject – said it was utterly foolish – despite the fact that five assorted dogs travelled everywhere with him in his car. Now, thirty-five years later, he is just as strongly in favour of keeping pets, though he now carries only one dog in his car. So, as I say, it was difficult to assess his reactions in this field and I refrained from following the little animal.

I was standing there when a young policeman came up to me.

'I've been watching that little dog begging among the stalls all morning,' he said. 'But like you, I haven't been able to get near him.'

'Yes, it's strange. He's obviously friendly, yet he's afraid. I wonder who owns him.'

'I reckon he's a stray, Mr Herriot. I'm interested in dogs myself and I fancy I know just about all of them around here. But this 'un's a stranger to me.'

I nodded. 'I bet you're right. So anything could have happened to him. He could have been ill-treated by somebody and run away, or he could have been dumped from a car.'

'Yes,' he replied. 'There's some lovely people around. It beats me how anybody can leave a helpless animal to fend for itself like that. I've had a few goes at catching him myself but it's no good.'

The memory stayed with me for the rest of the day and even when I lay in bed that night I was unable to dispel the disturbing image of the little brown creature wandering in a strange world, sitting up asking for help in the only way he knew.

＊

I was still a bachelor at that time and on the Friday night of the same week Siegfried and I were arraying ourselves in evening dress in preparation for the Hunt Ball at East Hirdsley, about ten miles away.

It was a tortuous business because those were the days of starched shirt fronts and stiff high collars and I kept hearing explosions of colourful language from Siegfried's room as he wrestled with his studs.

I was in an even worse plight because I had outgrown my suit and even when I had managed to secure the strangling collar I had to fight my way into the dinner jacket which nipped me cruelly under the arms. I had just managed to don the complete outfit and was trying out a few careful breaths when the phone rang.

It was the same young policeman I had been speaking to earlier in the week.

'We've got that dog round here, Mr Herriot. You know – the one that was begging in the market place.'

'Oh yes ? Somebody's managed to catch him, then ?'

There was a pause. 'No, not really. One of our men found him lying by the roadside about a mile out of town and brought him in. He's been in an accident.'

I told Siegfried. He looked at his watch. 'Always happens, doesn't it, James. Just when we're ready to go out. It's nine o'clock now and we should be on our way.' He thought for a moment. 'Anyway, slip round there and have a look and I'll wait for you. It would be better if we could go to this affair together.'

As I drove round to the police station I hoped fervently that there wouldn't be much to do. This Hunt Ball meant a lot to my boss because it would be a gathering of the horse-loving fraternity of the district and he would have a wonderful time just chatting and drinking with so many kindred spirits even though he hardly danced at all. Also, he maintained, it was good for business to meet the clients socially.

The kennels were at the bottom of a yard behind the station and the policeman led me down and opened one of the doors. The little dog was lying very still under the single electric bulb and when I bent and stroked the brown coat his tail stirred briefly among the straw of his bed.

'He can still manage a wag, anyway,' I said.

The policeman nodded. 'Aye, there's no doubt he's a good-natured little thing.'

I tried to examine him as much as possible without touching. I didn't want to hurt him and there was no saying what the extent of his injuries might be. But even at a glance certain things were obvious; he had multiple lacerations, one hind leg was crooked in the unmistakeable posture of a fracture and there was blood on his lips.

This could be from damaged teeth and I gently raised the head with a view to looking into his mouth. He was lying on his right side and as the head came round it was as though somebody had struck me in the face.

The right eye had been violently dislodged from its socket and it sprouted like some hideous growth from above the cheek bone, a great glistening orb with the eyelids tucked behind the white expanse of sclera.

I seemed to squat there for a long time, stunned by the obscenity, and as the seconds dragged by I looked into the little dog's face and he looked back at me – trustingly from one soft brown eye, glaring meaninglessly from the grotesque ball on the other side.

The policeman's voice broke my thoughts. 'He's a mess, isn't he?'

'Yes . . . yes . . . must have been struck by some vehicle – maybe dragged along by the look of all those wounds.'

'What d'you think, Mr Herriot?'

I knew what he meant. It was the sensible thing to ease this lost unwanted creature from the world. He was grieviously hurt and he didn't seem to belong to anybody. A quick overdose of anaesthetic – his troubles would be over and I'd be on my way to the dance.

But the policeman didn't say anything of the sort. Maybe, like me, he was looking into the soft depths of that one trusting eye.

I stood up quickly. 'Can I use your phone?'

At the other end of the line Siegfried's voice crackled with impatience. 'Hell, James, it's half-past nine! If we're going to this thing we've got to go now or we might as well not bother. A stray dog, badly injured. It doesn't sound such a great problem.'

'I know, Siegfried. I'm sorry to hold you up but I can't make up my mind. I wish you'd come round and tell me what you think.'

There was a silence then a long sigh. 'All right, James. See you in five minutes.'

He created a slight stir as he entered the station. Even in his casual working clothes Siegfried always managed to look distinguished, but as he swept into the station newly bathed and shaved, a camel coat thrown over the sparkling white shirt and black tie there was something ducal about him.

He drew respectful glances from the men sitting around, then my young policeman stepped forward.

'This way, sir,' he said, and we went back to the kennels.

Siegfried was silent as he crouched over the dog, looking him over as I had done without touching him. Then he carefully raised the head and the monstrous eye glared.

'My God!' he said softly, and at the sound of his voice the long fringed tail moved along the ground.

For a few seconds he stayed very still looking fixedly at the dog's face while in the silence, the whisking tail rustled the straw.

Then he straightened up. 'Let's get him round there,' he murmured.

In the surgery we anaesthetized the little animal and as he lay unconscious on the table we were able to examine him thoroughly. After a few minutes Siegfried stuffed his stethoscope into the pocket of his white coat and leaned both hands on the table.

'Luxated eyeball, fractured femur, umpteen deep lacerations, broken claws. There's enough here to keep us going till midnight, James.'

I didn't say anything.

My boss pulled the knot from his black tie and undid the front stud. He peeled off the stiff collar and hung it on the cross bar of the surgery lamp...

'By God, that's better,' he muttered, and began to lay out suture materials.

I looked at him across the table. 'How about the Hunt Ball ?'

'Oh bugger the Hunt Ball,' Siegfried said. 'Let's get busy.'

We were busy, too, for a long time. I hung up my collar next to my colleague's and we began on the eye. I know we both felt the same – we wanted to get rid of that horror before we did anything else.

I lubricated the great ball and pulled the eyelids apart while Siegfried gently manoeuvred it back into the orbital cavity. I sighed as everything slid out of sight, leaving only the cornea visible.

Siegfried chuckled with satisfaction. 'Looks like an eye again, doesn't it.' He seized an ophthalmoscope and peered into the depths.

'And there's no major damage – could be as good as new again. But we'll just stitch the lids together to protect it for a few days.'

The broken ends of the fractured tibia were badly displaced and we had to struggle to bring them into apposition before applying the plaster of paris. But at last we finished and started on the long job of stitching the many cuts and lacerations.

We worked separately for this, and for a long time it was quiet in the operating room except for the snip of scissors as we clipped the brown hair away from the wounds. I knew and Siegfried knew that we were almost certainly working without payment, but the most disturbing thought was that after all our efforts we might still have to put him down. He was still in the care of the police and if nobody claimed him within ten days it meant euthanasia. And if his late owners were really interested in his fate, why hadn't they tried to contact the police before now . . .

By the time we had completed our work and washed the instruments it was after midnight. Siegfried dropped the last suture needle into its tray and looked at the sleeping animal.

'I think he's beginning to come round,' he said. 'Let's take him through to the fire and we can have a drink while he recovers.'

We stretchered the dog through to the sitting room on a blanket and laid him on the rug before the brightly burning coals. My colleague reached a long arm up to the glass-fronted cabinet above the mantelpiece and pulled down the whisky bottle and two glasses. Drinks in hand, collarless, still in shirt sleeves, with our starched white fronts and braided evening trousers to remind us of the lost dance we lay back in our chairs on either side of the fireplace and between us our patient stretched peacefully.

He was a happier sight now. One eye was closed by the protecting stitches and his hind leg projected stiffly in its white cast, but he was tidy, cleaned up, cared for. He looked as though he belonged to somebody – but then there was a great big doubt about that.

It was nearly one o'clock in the morning and we were getting well down the bottle when the shaggy brown head began to move.

Siegfried leaned forward and touched one of the ears and immediately the tail flapped against the rug and a pink tongue lazily licked his fingers.

'What an absolutely grand little dog,' he murmured, but his voice had a distant quality. I knew he was worried too.

I took the stitches out of the eyelids two days after and was delighted to find a normal eye underneath.

The young policeman was as pleased as I was. 'Look at that!' he exclaimed. 'You'd never know anything had happened there.'

'Yes, it's done wonderfully well. All the swelling and inflammation has gone.' I hesitated for a moment. 'Has anybody inquired about him ?'

He shook his head. 'Nothing yet. But there's another eight days to go and we're taking good care of him here.'

I visited the police station several times and the little animal greeted me with undisguised joy, all his fear gone, standing upright against my legs on his plastered limb, his tail swishing.

But all the time my sense of foreboding increased, and on the tenth day I made my way almost with dread to the police kennels. I had heard nothing. My course of action seemed inevitable. Putting down old or hopelessly ill dogs was often an act of mercy but when it was a young healthy dog it was terrible. I hated it, but it was one of those things veterinary surgeons had to do.

The young policeman was standing in the doorway.

'Still no news ?' I asked, and he shook his head.

I went past him into the kennel and the shaggy little creature stood up against my legs as before, laughing into my face, mouth open, eyes shining.

I turned away quickly. I'd have to do this right now or I'd never do it.

'Mr Herriot.' The policeman put his hand on my arm. 'I think I'll take him.'

'You ?' I stared at him.

'Aye, that's right. We got a lot o' stray dogs in here and though I feel sorry for them you can't give them all a home, can you?'

'No, you can't,' I said. 'I have the same problem.'

He nodded slowly. 'But somehow this 'un's different, and it seems to me he's just come at the right time. I have two little girls and they've been at me for a bit to get 'em a dog. This little bloke looks just right for the job.'

Warm relief began to ebb through me. 'I couldn't agree more. He's the soul of good nature. I bet he'll be wonderful with children.'

'Good. That's settled then. I thought I'd ask your advice first.' He smiled happily.

I looked at him as though I had never seen him before. 'What's your name?'

'Phelps,' he replied. 'PC Phelps.'

He was a good-looking young fellow, clear-skinned, with cheerful blue eyes and a solid dependable look about him. I had to fight against an impulse to wring his hand and thump him on the back. But I managed to preserve the professional exterior.

'Well, that's fine.' I bent and stroked the little dog. 'Don't forget to bring him along to the surgery in ten days for removal of the stitches, and we'll have to get that plaster off in about a month.'

It was Siegfried who took out the stitches, and I didn't see our patient again until four weeks later.

PC Phelps had his little girls, aged four and six, with him as well as the dog.

'You said the plaster ought to come off about now,' he said, and I nodded.

He looked down at the children. 'Well, come on, you two, lift him on the table.'

Eagerly the little girls put their arms around their new pet and as they hoisted him the tail wagged furiously and the wide mouth panted in delight.

'Looks as though he's been a success,' I said.

He smiled. 'That's an understatement. He's perfect with these two. I can't tell you what pleasure he's given us. He's one of the family.'

I got out my little saw and began to hack at the plaster.

'It's worked both ways, I should say. A dog loves a secure home.'

'Well, he couldn't be more secure.' He ran his hand along the brown coat and laughed as he addressed the little dog. 'That's what you get for begging among the stalls on market day, my lad. You're in the hands of the law now.'

8

When I entered the RAF I had a secret fear. All my life I have suffered from vertigo and even now I have only to look down from the smallest height to be engulfed by that dreadful dizziness and panic. What would I feel, then, when I started to fly?

As it turned out, I felt nothing. I could gaze downwards from the open cockpit through thousands of feet of space without a qualm, so my fear was groundless.

I had my fears in veterinary practice, too, and in the early days the thing which raised the greatest terror in my breast was the Ministry of Agriculture.

An extraordinary statement, perhaps, but true. It was the clerical side that scared me – all those forms. As to the practical Ministry work itself, I felt in all modesty that I was quite good at it. My thoughts often turned back to all the tuberculin testing I used to do – clipping a clean little area from just the right place in the cow's neck, inserting the needle into the thickness of the skin and injecting one tenth of a cc of tuberculin.

It was on Mr Hill's farm, and I watched the satisfactory intradermal 'pea' rise up under my needle. That was the way it should be, and when it came up like that you knew you were really doing your job and testing the animal for tuberculosis.

'That 'un's number sixty-five,' the farmer said, then a slightly injured look spread over his face as I checked the number in the ear.

'You're wastin' your time, Mr Herriot. I 'ave the whole list, all in t'correct order. Wrote it out special for you so you could take it away with you.'

I had my doubts. All farmers were convinced that their herd records were flawless but I had been caught out before. I seemed to have the gift of making every possible clerical mistake and I didn't need any help from the farmers.

But still . . . it was tempting. I looked at the long list of figures dangling from the horny fingers. If I accepted it I would save a lot of time. There were still more than fifty animals to test here and I had to get through two more herds before lunch time.

I looked at my watch. Damn! I was well behind my programme and I felt the old stab of frustration.

'Right, Mr Hill, I'll take it and thank you very much.' I stuffed the sheet of paper into my pocket and began to move along the byre, clipping and injecting at top speed.

A week later the dread words leaped out at me from the open day book. 'Ring Min.' The cryptic phrase in Miss Harbottle's writing had the power to freeze my blood quicker than anything else. It meant simply that I had to telephone the Ministry of Agriculture office, and whenever our secretary wrote those words in the book it meant that I was in trouble again. I extended a trembling hand towards the receiver.

As always, Kitty Pattison answered my call and I could detect the note of pity in her voice. She was the attractive girl in charge of the office staff and she knew all about my misdemeanours. In fact when it was something very trivial she sometimes brought it to my attention herself, but when I had really dropped a large brick I was dealt with by the boss, Charles Harcourt, the Divisional Inspector.

'Ah, Mr Herriot,' Kitty said lightly. I knew she sympathized with me but she couldn't do a thing about it. 'Mr Harcourt wants a word with you.'

There it was. The terrible sentence that always set my heart thumping.

'Thank you,' I said huskily, and waited an eternity as the phone was switched through.

'Herriot!' The booming voice made me jump.

I swallowed. 'Good morning Mr Harcourt. How are you ?'

'I'll tell you how I am, I'm bloody annoyed!' I could imagine vividly the handsome, high-coloured, choleric face flushing deeper, the greenish eyes glaring. 'In fact I'm hopping bloody mad!'

'Oh.'

'It's no use saying "oh". That's what you said the last time when you tested that cow of Frankland's that had been dead for two years! That was very clever – I don't know how you managed it. Now I've been going over your test at Hill's of High View and there are two cows here that you've tested – numbers 74 and 103. Now our records show that he sold both of them at Brawton Auction Mart six months ago, so you've performed another miracle.'

'I'm sorry . . .'

'Please don't be sorry, it's bloody marvellous how you do it. I have all the figures here – skin measurements, the lot. I see you found they were both thin-skinned animals even though they were about fifteen miles away at the time. Clever stuff!'

'Well I . . .'

'All right, Herriot, I'll dispense with the comedy. I'm going to tell you once more; for the last time, and I hope you're listening.' He paused and I could almost see the big shoulders hunching as he barked into the phone. '*Look in the bloody ears in future!*'

I broke into a rapid gabble. 'I will indeed, Mr Harcourt, I assure you from now on . . .'

'All right, all right, but there's something else.'

'Something else?'

'Yes, I'm not finished yet.' The voice took on a great weariness. 'Can I ask you to cast your mind back to that cow you took under the TB order from Wilson of Low Parks?'

I dug my nails into my palm. We were heading for deep water. 'Yes – I remember it.'

'Well now, Herriot, lad, do you remember a little chat we had about the forms?' Charles was trying to be patient, because he was a decent man, but it was costing him dearly. 'Didn't anything I told you sink in?'

'Well, yes, of course.'

'Then why, why didn't you send me a receipt for slaughter?'

'Receipt for . . . didn't I . . . ?'

'No, you didn't,' he said. 'And honestly I can't understand it.

I went over it with you step by step last time when you forgot to forward a copy of the valuation agreement.'

'Oh dear, I really am sorry.'

A deep sigh came from the other end. 'And there's nothing to it.' He paused. 'Tell you what we'll do. Let's go over the procedure once more, shall we?'

'Yes, by all means.'

'Very well,' he said. 'First of all, when you find an infected animal you serve B 205 DT, Form A, which is the notice requiring detention and isolation of the animal. Next,' and I could hear the slap of finger on palm as he enumerated his points, 'next, there is B 207 DT, Form C, Notice of intended slaughter. Then B 208 DT, Form D, Post-mortem Certificate. Then B 196 DT, Veterinary Inspector's report. Then B 209 DT, Valuation agreement, and in cases where the owner objects, there is B 213 DT, Appointment of valuer. Then we have B 212 DT, Notice to owner of time and place of slaughter, followed by B 227 DT, Receipt for animal for slaughter, and finally B 230 DT, Notice requiring cleansing and disinfection. Dammit, a child could understand that. It's perfectly simple, isn't it?'

'Yes, yes, certainly, absolutely.' It wasn't simple to me, but I didn't mention the fact. He had calmed down nicely and I didn't want to inflame him again.

'Well thank you, Mr Harcourt,' I said. 'I'll see it doesn't happen again.' I put down the receiver with the feeling that things could have turned out a lot worse, but for all that my nerves didn't stop jangling for some time. The trouble was that the Ministry work was desperately important to general practitioners. In fact, in those precarious days it was the main rent payer.

This business of the Tuberculosis Order. When a veterinary surgeon came upon a cow with open TB it was his duty to see that the animal was slaughtered immediately because its milk could be a danger to the public. That sounds easy, but unfortunately the law insisted that the demise of each unhappy creature be commemorated by a confetti-like shower of the doom-laden forms.

It wasn't just that there were so many of these forms, but they had to be sent to an amazing variety of people. Sometimes I used to think that there were very few people in England who didn't get one. Apart from Charles Harcourt, other recipients included the farmer concerned, the police, the Head Office of the Ministry, the knacker man, the local authority. I nearly always managed to forget one of them. I used to have nightmares about standing in the middle of the market place, throwing the forms around me at the passers-by and laughing hysterically.

Looking back, I can hardly believe that for all this wear and tear on the nervous system the payment was one guinea plus ten and sixpence for the post-mortem.

It was a mere two days after my interview with the Divisional Inspector that I had to take another cow under the TB Order. When I came to fill in the forms I sat at the surgery desk in a dither of apprehension, going over them again and again, laying them out side by side and enclosing them one by one in their various envelopes. This time there must be no mistake.

I took them over to the post myself and uttered a silent prayer as I dropped them into the box. Charles would have them the following morning, and I would soon know if I had done it again. When two days passed without incident I felt I was safe, but midway through the third morning I dropped in at the surgery and read the message in letters of fire. 'RING MIN!'

Kitty Pattison sounded strained. She didn't even try to appear casual. 'Oh yes, Mr Herriot,' she said hurriedly. 'Mr Harcourt asked me to call you. I'm putting you through now.'

My heart almost stopped as I waited for the familiar bellow, but when the quiet voice came on the line it frightened me even more.

'Good morning, Herriot.' Charles was curt and impersonal. 'I'd like to discuss that last cow you took under the Order.'

'Oh yes?' I croaked.

'But not over the telephone. I want to see you here in the office.'

'In the . . . the office?'

'Yes, right away if you can.'

I put down the phone and went out to the car with my knees knocking. Charles Harcourt was really upset this time. There was a kind of restrained fury in his words, and this business of going to the office – that was reserved for serious transgressions.

Twenty minutes later my footsteps echoed in the corridor of

the Ministry building. Marching stiffly like a condemned man I passed the windows where I could see the typists at work, then I read 'Divisional Inspector' on the door at the end.

I took one long shuddering breath, then knocked.

'Come in.' The voice was still quiet and controlled.

Charles looked up unsmilingly from his desk as I entered. He motioned me to a chair and directed a cold stare at me.

'Herriot,' he said unemotionally. 'You're really on the carpet this time.'

Charles had been a major in the Punjabi Rifles and he was very much the Indian Army officer at this moment. A fine looking man, clear-skinned and ruddy, with massive cheek bones above a powerful jaw. Looking at the dangerously glinting eyes it struck me that only a fool would trifle with somebody like him – and I had a nasty feeling that I had been trifling.

Dry-mouthed, I waited.

'You know, Herriot,' he went on. 'After our last telephone conversation about TB forms I thought you might give me a little peace.'

'Peace . . . ?'

'Yes, yes, it was silly of me, I know, but when I took all that time to go over the procedure with you I actually thought you were listening.'

'Oh I was, I was!'

'You were ? Oh good.' He gave me a mirthless smile. 'Then I suppose it was even more foolish of me to expect you to act upon my instructions. In my innocence I thought you cared about what I was telling you.'

'Mr Harcourt, believe me, I do care, I . . .'

'*Then why*,' he bawled without warning, bringing his great hand flailing down on the desk with a crash that made pens and inkwells dance, '*why the bloody hell do you keep making a balls of it ?*'

I resisted a strong impulse to run away. 'Making a . . . I don't quite understand.'

'You don't ?' He kept up his pounding on the desk. 'Well I'll tell you. One of my veterinary officers was on that farm, and he found that you hadn't served a Notice of cleansing and disinfection!'

'Is that so?'

'Yes, it bloody well is so! You didn't give one to the farmer but you sent one to me. Maybe you want me to go and disinfect the place, is that it? Would you like me to slip along there and get busy with a hosepipe – I'll go now if it'll make you feel any happier!'

'Oh no, no, no . . . no.'

He was apparently not satisfied with the thunderous noise he was making because he began to use both hands, bringing them down simultaneously with sickening force on the wood while he glared wildly.

'Herriot!' he shouted. 'There's just one thing I want to know from you – do you want this bloody work or don't you? Just say the word and I'll give it to another practice and then maybe we'd both be able to live a quiet life!'

'Please, Mr Harcourt, I give you my word, I . . . we . . . we do want the work very much.' And I meant it with all my heart.

The big man slumped back in his chair and regarded me for a few moments in silence. Then he glanced at his wrist watch.

'Ten past twelve,' he murmured. 'Just time to have a beer at the Red Lion before lunch.'

In the pub lounge he took a long pull at his glass, placed it carefully on the table in front of him, then turned to me with a touch of weariness.

'You know, Herriot, I do wish you'd stop doing this sort of thing. It takes it out of me.'

I believed him. His face had lost a little of its colour and his hand trembled slightly as he raised his glass again.

'I'm truly sorry, Mr Harcourt, I don't know how it happened. I did try to get it right this time and I'll do my best to avoid troubling you in future.'

He nodded a few times, then clapped me on the shoulder. 'Good, good – let's just have one more.'

He moved over to the bar, brought back the drinks then fished out a brown paper parcel from his pocket.

'Little wedding present, Herriot. Understand you're getting married soon – this is from my missus and me with our best wishes.'

I didn't know what to say. I fumbled the wrapping away and uncovered a small square barometer.

Shame engulfed me as I muttered a few words of thanks. This man was the head of the Ministry in the area while I was the newest and lowest of his minions. Not only that, but I was pretty sure I caused him more trouble than all the others put together – I was like a hair shirt to him. There was no earthly reason why he should give me a barometer.

This last experience deepened my dread of form filling to the extent that I hoped it would be a long time before I encountered another tuberculous animal, but fate decreed that I had some concentrated days of clinical inspections and it was with a feeling of inevitability that I surveyed Mr Moverley's Ayrshire cow.

It was the soft cough which made me stop and look at her more closely, and as I studied her my spirits sank. This was another one. The skin stretched tightly over the bony frame, the slightly accelerated respirations and that deep careful cough. Mercifully you don't see cows like that now, but in those days they were all too common.

I moved along her side and examined the wall in front of her. The tell-tale blobs of sputum were clearly visible on the rough stones and I quickly lifted a sample and smeared it on a glass slide.

Back at the surgery I stained the smear by Ziehl-Nielson's method and pushed the slide under the microscope. The red clumps of tubercle bacilli lay among the scattered cells, tiny, iridescent and deadly. I hadn't really needed the grim proof but it was there.

Mr Moverley was not amused when I told him next morning the animal would have to be slaughtered.

'It's nobbut got a bit of a chill,' he grunted. The farmers were never pleased when one of their milk producers was removed by a petty bureaucrat like me. 'But ah suppose it's no use arguin'.'

'I assure you, Mr Moverley, there's no doubt about it. I examined that sample last night and . . .'

'Oh, never mind about that.' The farmer waved an impatient hand. 'If t'bloody government says me cow's got to go she's got to go. But ah get compensation, don't I ?'

'Yes, you do.'

'How much ?'

I thought rapidly. The rules stated that the animal be valued as if it were up for sale in the open market in its present condition. The minimum was five pounds and there was no doubt that this emaciated cow came into that category.

'The statutory value is five pounds,' I said.

'Shit!' replied Mr Moverley.

'We can appoint a valuer if you don't agree.'

'Oh 'ell, let's get t'job over with.' He was clearly disgusted and I thought it imprudent to tell him that he would only get a proportion of the five pounds, depending on the post-mortem.

'Very well,' I said. 'I'll tell Jeff Mallock to collect her as soon as possible.'

The fact that I was unpopular with Mr Moverley didn't worry me as much as the prospect of dealing with the dreaded forms. The very thought of sending another batch winging hopefully on its way to Charles Harcourt brought me out in a sweat.

Then I had a flash of inspiration. Such things don't often happen to me, but this struck me as brilliant. I wouldn't send off the forms till I'd had them vetted by Kitty Pattison.

I couldn't wait to get the plan under way. Almost gleefully I laid the papers out in a long row, signed them and laid them by their envelopes, ready for their varied journeys. Then I phoned the Ministry office.

Kitty was patient and kind. I am sure she realized that I did my work conscientiously but that I was a clerical numbskull and she sympathized.

When I had finished going through the list she congratulated me. 'Well done, Mr Herriot, you've got them right this time! All you need now is the knacker man's signature and your post-mortem report and you're home and dry.'

'Bless you, Kitty,' I said. 'You've made my day.'

And she had. The airy sensation of relief was tremendous. The knowledge that there would be no come-back from Charles this time was like the sun bursting through dark clouds. I felt like singing as I went round to Mallock's yard and arranged with him to pick up the cow.

'Have her ready for me to inspect tomorrow, Jeff,' I said, and went on my way with a light heart.

I couldn't understand it when Mr Moverley waved me down

from his farm gate next day. As I drew up I could see he was extremely agitated.

'Hey!' he cried. 'Ah've just got back from the market and my missus tells me Mallock's been!'

I smiled. 'That's right, Mr Moverley. Remember I told you I was going to send him round for your cow.'

'Aye, ah know all about that!' He paused and glared at me. 'But he's took the wrong one!'

'Wrong . . . wrong what?'

'Wrong cow, that's what! He's off wi' the best cow in me herd. Pedigree Ayrshire – ah bought 'er in Dumfries last week and they only delivered 'er this mornin'.'

Horror drove through me in a freezing wave. I had told the knacker man to collect the Ayrshire which would be isolated in the loose box in the yard. The new animal would be in a box, too, after her arrival. I could see Jeff and his man leading her up the ramp into his wagon with a dreadful clarity.

'This is your responsibility, tha knaws!' The farmer waved a threatening finger. 'If he kills me good cow you'll 'ave to answer for it!'

He didn't have to tell me. I'd have to answer for it to a lot of people, including Charles Harcourt.

'Get on the phone to the knacker yard right away!' I gasped.

The farmer waved his arms about. 'Ah've tried that and there's no reply. Ah tell ye he'll shoot 'er afore we can stop 'im. Do you know how much ah paid for that cow?'

'Never mind about that! Which way did he go?'

'T'missus said he went towards Grampton – about ten minutes ago.'

I started my engine. 'He'll maybe be picking up other beasts – I'll go after him.'

Teeth clenched, eyes popping, I roared along the Grampton road. The enormity of this latest catastrophe was almost more than I could assimilate. The wrong form was bad enough, but the wrong cow was unthinkable. But it had happened. Charles would crucify me this time. He was a good bloke but he would have no option, because the higher-ups in the Ministry would get wind of an immortal boner like this and they would howl for blood.

Feverishly but vainly I scanned each farm entrance in Grampton village as I shot through, and when I saw the open country-side ahead of me again the tension was almost unbearable. I was telling myself that the whole thing was hopeless when in the far distance above a row of trees I spotted the familiar top of Mallock's wagon.

It was a high, wooden-sided vehicle and I couldn't mistake it. Repressing a shout of triumph I put my foot on the boards and set off in that direction with the fanatical zeal of the hunter. But it was a long way off and I hadn't travelled a mile before I realized I had lost it.

Over the years many things have stayed in my memory, but the Great Cow Chase is engraven deeper than most. The sheer terror I felt is vivid to this day. I kept sighting the wagon among the maze of lanes and side roads, but by the time I had cut across country my quarry had disappeared behind a hillside or dipped into one of the many hollows in the wide vista. I was constantly deceived by the fact that I expected him to be turning towards Darrowby after passing through a village, but he never did. Clearly he had other business on the way.

The whole thing seemed to last a very long time and there was no fun in it for me. I was gripped throughout by a cold dread, and the violent swings – the alternating scents of hope and despair – were wearing to the point of exhaustion. I was utterly drained when at last I saw the tall lorry rocking along a straight road in front of me.

I had him now! Forcing my little car to the limit, I drew abreast of him, sounding my horn repeatedly till he stopped. Breathlessly I pulled up in front of him and ran round to offer my explanations. But as I looked up into the driver's cab my eager smile vanished. It wasn't Jeff Mallock at all. I had been following the wrong man.

It was the 'ket feller'. He had exactly the same type of wagon as Mallock and he went round a wide area of Yorkshire picking up the nameless odds and ends of the dead animals which even the knacker men didn't want. It was a strange job and he was a strange-looking man. The oddly piercing eyes glittered uncannily from under a tattered army peaked cap.

'Wot's up, guvnor?' He removed a cigarette from his mouth and spat companionably into the roadway.

My throat was tight. 'I – I'm sorry. I thought you were Jeff Mallock.'

The eyes did not change expression, but the corner of his mouth twitched briefly. 'If tha wants Jeff he'll be back at his yard now, ah reckon.' He spat again and replaced his cigarette.

I nodded dully. Jeff would be there now all right – long ago. I had been chasing the wrong wagon for about an hour and that cow would be dead and hanging up on hooks at this moment. The knacker man was a fast and skilful worker and wasted no time when he got back with his beasts.

'Well, ah'm off 'ome now,' the ket feller said. 'So long, boss.' He winked at me, started his engine and the big vehicle rumbled away.

I trailed back to my car. There was no hurry now. And strangely, now that all was lost my mood relaxed. In fact, as I drove away, a great calm settled on me and I began to assess my future with cool objectivity. I would be drummed out of the Ministry's service for sure, and idly I wondered if they had any special ceremony for the occasion – perhaps a ritual stripping of the Panel Certificates or something of the sort.

I tried to put away the thought that more than the Ministry would be interested in my latest exploit. How about the Royal College ? Did they strike you off for something like this ? Well, it was possible, and in my serene state of mind I toyed with the possibilities of alternative avenues of employment. I had often thought it must be fun to run a secondhand book shop and now that I began to consider it seriously I felt sure there was an opening for one in Darrowby. I experienced a comfortable glow at the vision of myself sitting under the rows of dusty volumes, pulling one down from the shelf when I felt like it or maybe just looking out into the street through the window from my safe little world where there were no forms or telephones or messages saying, 'Ring Min.'

In Darrowby I drove round without haste to the knacker yard. I left my car outside the grim little building with the black smoke drifting from its chimney. I pulled back the sliding door and saw Jeff seated at his ease on a pile of cow hides, holding a slice of apple pie in blood-stained fingers. And, ah yes, there, just behind him hung the two great sides of beef and on the floor, the lungs, bowels and other viscera – the sad remnants of Mr Moverley's pedigree Ayrshire.

'Hello, Jeff,' I said.

'Now then, Mr Herriot.' He gave me the beatific smile which mirrored his personality so well. 'Ah'm just havin' a little snack. I allus like a bite about this time.' He sank his teeth into the pie and chewed appreciatively.

'So I see.' I sorrowfully scanned the hanging carcass. Just dog meat and not even much of that. Ayrshires were never very fat. I was wondering how to break the news to him when he spoke again.

'Ah'm sorry you've caught me out this time, Mr Herriot,' he said, reaching for a greasy mug of tea.

'What do you mean?'

'Well, I allus reckon to have t'beast dressed and ready for you but you've come a bit early.'

I stared at him. 'But . . . everything's here, surely.' I waved a hand around me.

'Nay, nay, that's not 'er.'

'You mean . . . that isn't the cow from Moverley's.'

'That's right.' He took a long draught from the mug and wiped his mouth with the back of his hand. 'I 'ad to do this 'un first. Moverley's cow's still in t'wagon out at the back.'

'Alive?'

He looked mildly surprised. 'Aye, of course. She's never had a finger on 'er. Nice cow for a screw, too.'

I could have fainted with relief. 'She's no screw, Jeff. That's the wrong cow you've got there?'

'Wrong cow?' Nothing ever startled him but he obviously desired more information. I told him the whole story.

When I had finished, his shoulders began to shake gently and the beautiful clear eyes twinkled in the pink face.

'Well, that's a licker,' he murmured, and continued to laugh gently. There was nothing immoderate in his mirth and indeed nothing I had said disturbed him in the least. The fact that he had wasted his journey or that the farmer might be annoyed was of no moment to him.

Again, looking at Jeff Mallock, it struck me, as many times before, that there was nothing like à lifetime of dabbling among diseased carcasses and lethal bacteria for breeding tranquillity of mind.

'You'll slip back and change the cow?' I said.

'Aye, in a minute or two. There's nowt spoilin'. Ah never likes to hurry me grub.' He belched contentedly. 'And how about you, Mr Herriot? You could do with summat to keep your strength up.' He produced another mug and broke off a generous wedge of pie which he offered to me.

'No ... no ... er ... no, thank you, Jeff. It's kind of you, but no ... no ... not just now.'

He shrugged his shoulders and smiled as he stretched an arm for his pipe which was balanced on a sheep's skull. Flicking away some shreds of stray tissue from the stem he applied a match and settled down blissfully on the hides.

'I'll see ye later, then,' he said. 'Come round tonight and everything'll be ready for you.' He closed his eyes and again his shoulders quivered. 'Ah'd better get the right 'un this time.'

It must be more than twenty years since I took a cow under the TB Order, because the clinical cases so rarely exist now. 'Ring Min' no longer has the power to chill my blood, and the dread forms which scarred my soul lie unused and yellowing in the bottom of a drawer.

All these things have gone from my life. Charles Harcourt has gone too, but I think of him every day when I look at the little barometer which still hangs on my wall.

9

'Oh Mr Herriot!' Mrs Ridge said delightedly. 'Somebody stole our car last night.' She looked at me with a radiant smile.

I was lying on my bed in the barrack hut at Winkfield listening to somebody on the radio adjuring people to immobilize their cars in wartime when this lady's strange remark bubbled back from my veterinary days.

I stopped in the doorway of her house. 'Mrs Ridge, I'm terribly sorry. How . . . ?'

'Yes, yes, oh I can't wait to tell you!' Her voice trembled with excitement and joy. 'There must have been some prowlers around here last night, and I'm such a silly about leaving the car unlocked.'

'I see . . . how unfortunate.'

'But do come in,' she giggled. 'Forgive me for keeping you standing on the step, but I'm all of a dither!'

I went past her into the lounge. 'Well, it's very understandable. It must have been quite a shock.'

'Shock? Oh, but you don't see what I mean. It's wonderful!'

'Eh?'

'Yes, of course!' She clasped her hands and looked up at the ceiling. 'Do you know what happened?'

'Well, yes,' I said. 'You've just told me.'

'No, I haven't told you half.'

'You haven't?'

'No, but do sit down. I know you'll want to hear all about it.'

To explain this I have to go back ten days to the afternoon when Mrs Ridge ran tearfully up the steps of Skeldale House.

'My little dog's had an accident,' she gasped.

I looked past her. 'Where is he?'

'In the car. I didn't know whether I should move him.'

I crossed the pavement and opened the door. Her Cairn terrier, Joshua, lay very still on a blanket on the back seat.

'What happened?' I asked.

She put a hand over her eyes. 'Oh, it was terrible. You know he often plays in the farmer's field opposite our house – well, about half an hour ago he started to chase a rabbit and ran under the wheels of a tractor.'

I looked from her face to the motionless animal and back again. 'Did the wheels go over him?'

She nodded as the tears streamed down her cheeks.

I took her by the arm. 'Mrs Ridge, this is important. Are you absolutely sure that wheel passed right over his body?'

'Yes, I am – quite certain. I saw it happen. I couldn't believe he'd be alive when I ran to pick him up.' She took a long breath. 'I don't suppose he can live after that, can he?'

I didn't want to depress her but it seemed impossible that a small dog like this could survive being crushed under that great weight. Massive internal damage would be inevitable apart altogether from broken bones. It was sad to see the little sandy form lying still and unheeding when I had watched him so often running and leaping in the fields.

'Let's have a look at him,' I said.

I climbed into the car and sat down on the seat beside him. With the utmost care I felt my way over the limbs, expecting every moment to feel the crepitus which would indicate a fracture. I put my hand underneath him very slowly, supporting his weight every inch of the way. The only time Joshua showed any reaction was when I moved the pelvic girdle.

The best sign of all was the pinkness of the mucous membranes of eye and mouth and I turned to Mrs Ridge rather more hopefully.

'Miraculously he doesn't seem to have an internal haemorrhage and there are no limb bones broken. I'm pretty sure he has a fractured pelvis, but that's not so bad.'

She drew her fingers over the smears on her cheeks and looked at me, wide-eyed. 'You really think he has a chance?'

'Well, I don't want to raise your hopes unduly, but at this moment I can't find any sign of severe injury.'

'But it doesn't seem possible.'

I shrugged. 'I agree, it doesn't, but if he has got away with it I can only think it was because he was on soft ground which yielded as the wheel squeezed him down. Anyway, let's get him X-rayed to make sure.'

At that time, in common with most large animal practices, we didn't have an X-ray machine, but the local hospital helped us out in times of need. I took Joshua round there and the picture confirmed my diagnosis of pelvic fracture.

'There's not much I can do,' I said to his mistress. 'This type of injury usually heals itself. He'll probably have difficulty in standing on his hind legs for a while and for several weeks he'll be weak in the rear end, but with rest and time he ought to recover.'

'Oh, marvellous!' She watched me place the little animal back on the car seat. 'I suppose it's just a matter of waiting, then?'

'That's what I hope.'

My fears that Joshua might have some internal damage were finally allayed when I saw him two days later. His membranes were a rich deep pink and all natural functions were operating.

Mrs Ridge, however, was still worried. 'He's such a sorrowful little thing,' she said. 'Just look at him – he's lifeless.'

'Well you know he must be bruised and sore after that squashing he had. And he was very shocked, too. You must be patient.'

As I spoke, the little dog stood up, wobbled a few feet across the carpet and flopped down again. He showed no interest in me or his surroundings.

Before I left I gave his mistress some salicylate tablets to give him. 'These will ease his discomfort,' I said. 'Let me know if he doesn't improve.'

She did let me know – within forty-eight hours. 'I wish you'd come and see Joshua again,' she said on the phone. 'I'm not at all happy about him."

The little animal was as before. I looked down at him as he lay dejectedly on the rug, head on his paws, looking into the fireplace.

'Come on, Joshua, old lad,' I said. 'You must be feeling better now.' I bent and rubbed my fingers along the wiry coat, but neither word or gesture made an impression. I might as well not have been there.

Mrs Ridge turned to me worriedly. 'That's what he's like all the time. And you know how he is normally.'

'Yes, he's always been a ball of fire.' Again I recalled him jumping round my legs, gazing up at me eagerly. 'It's very strange.'

'And another thing,' she went on. 'He never utters a sound. And you know, that worries me more than anything because he's always been such a good little watch dog. We used to hear him barking when the early post came, he barked at the milk boy, the dustman, everybody. He was never a yappy dog, but he let us know when anybody was around.'

'Yes . . .' That was another thing I remembered. The tumult of sound from within whenever I rang the door bell.

'And now there's just this dreadful silence. People come and go but he never even looks up.' She shook her head slowly. 'Oh, if only he'd bark! Just once! I think it would mean he was getting better.'

'It probably would,' I said.

'Is there something else wrong with him, do you think?' she asked.

I thought for a moment or two. 'No, I'm convinced there isn't. Not physically, anyway. He's had a tremendous fright and he has withdrawn within himself. He'll come out of it in time.'

As I left I had the feeling I was trying to convince myself as much as Mrs Ridge. And as, over the next few days, she kept phoning me with bad reports about the little dog my confidence began to ebb.

It was a week after the accident that she begged me to come to the house again. Joshua was unchanged. Apathetic, tail tucked down, sad-eyed – and still soundless.

His mistress was obviously under strain.

'Mr Herriot,' she said. 'What are we going to do? I can't sleep for thinking about him.'

I produced stethoscope and thermometer and examined the little animal again. Then I palpated him thoroughly from head to tail. When I had finished I squatted on the rug and looked up at Mrs Ridge.

'I can't find anything new. You'll just have to be patient.'

'But that's what you said before, and I feel I can't go on much longer like this.'

'Still no barking?'

She shook her head. 'No, and that's what I'm waiting for. He eats a little, walks around a little, but we never hear a sound from him. I know I'd stop worrying if I heard him bark, just once, but otherwise I have a horrible feeling he's going to die . . .'

*

I had hoped that my next visit would be more cheerful but though I was greatly relieved at Mrs Ridge's high spirits I was surprised, too.

I sat down in one of the comfortable chairs in the lounge.

'Well, I hope you'll soon recover your car,' I said.

She waved a hand negligently. 'Oh, it'll turn up somewhere, I'm sure.'

'But still – you must be very upset.'

'Upset? Not a bit! I'm so happy!'

'Happy? About losing the car . . . ?'

'No, not about that. About Joshua.'

'Joshua?'

'Yes.' She sat down in the chair opposite and leaned forward. 'Do you know what he did when those people were driving the car away?'

'No, tell me.'

'He *barked*, Mr Herriot! Joshua *barked*!'

10

The food was so good at the Winkfield flying school that it was said that those airmen whose homes were within visiting distance wouldn't take a day's leave because they might miss some culinary speciality. Difficult to believe, maybe, but I often think that few people in wartime Britain fared as well as the handful of young men in the scatter of wooden huts on that flat green stretch outside Windsor.

It wasn't as though we had a French chef, either. The cooking was done by two grizzled old men – civilians who wore cloth caps and smoked pipes and went about their business with unsmiling taciturnity.

It was rumoured that they were two ex-army cooks from the First World War, but whatever their origins they were artists. In their hands, simple stews and pies assumed a new significance and it was possible to rhapsodize even over the perfect flouriness of their potatoes.

So it was surprising when at lunchtime my neighbour on the left threw down his spoon, pushed away his plate and groaned. We ate on trestle tables, sitting in rows on long forms, and I was right up against the young man.

'What's wrong?' I asked. 'This apple dumpling is terrific.'

'Ah, it's not the grub.' He buried his face in his hands for a few seconds then looked at me with tortured eyes. 'I've been doing circuits and bumps this morning with Routledge and he's torn the knackers off me – all the time, it never stopped.'

Suddenly my own meal lost some of its flavour. I knew just what he meant. FO Woodham did the same to me.

He gave me another despairing glance, then stared straight ahead.

'I know one thing, Jim. I'll never make a bloody pilot.'

His words sent a chill through me. He was voicing the conviction which had been gradually growing in me. I never seemed to make any progress – whatever I did was wrong, and I was losing heart. Like all the others I was hoping to be graded pilot, but after every session with FO Woodham the idea of ever flying an aeroplane all on my own seemed more and more ludicrous. And I had another date with him at 2 p.m.

He was as quiet and charming as ever when I met him – till we got up into the sky and the shouting started again.

'Relax! For heavens sake, relax!' or 'Watch your height! Where the hell d'you think you're going?' or 'Didn't I tell you to centralize the stick? Are you bloody deaf or something?' And finally, after the first circuit when we juddered to a halt on the grass. 'That was an absolutely bloody ropy landing! Take off again!'

On the second circuit he fell strangely silent. And though I should have felt relieved I found something ominous in the unaccustomed peace. It could mean only one thing – he had finally given me up as a bad job. When we landed he told me to switch off the engine and climbed out of the rear cockpit. I was about to unbuckle my straps and follow him when he signalled me to remain in my seat.

'Stay where you are,' he said. 'You can take her up now.'

I stared down at him through my goggles. 'What ... ?'

'I said take her up.'

'You mean, on my own ... ? Go solo ... ?'

'Yes, of course. Come and see me in the flight hut after you've landed and taxied in.' He turned and walked away over the green. He didn't look back.

After a few minutes a fitter came over to where I sat trembling in my seat. He spat on the turf then looked at me with deep distaste.

'Look, mate,' he said. 'That's a — good aircraft you've got there.'

I nodded agreement.

'Well I don't want it — well smashed up, okay ?'

'Okay.'

He gave me a final disgusted glance, then went round to the propeller.

Panic-stricken though I was, I did not forget the cockpit drill which had been dinned in to me so often. I never thought I'd have to use it in earnest but now I automatically tested the controls – rudder, ailerons and elevator. Fuel on, switch off, throttle closed, then switch on, throttle slightly open.

'Contact!' I cried.

The fitter swung the propeller and the engine roared. I pushed the throttle full open and the Tiger Moth began to bump its way over the grass. As we gathered speed I eased the stick forward to lift the tail, then as I pulled it back again the bumping stopped and we climbed smoothly into the air with the long dining hut at the end of the airfield flashing away beneath.

I was gripped by exhilaration and triumph. The impossible had happened. I was up here on my own, flying, really flying at last. I had been so certain of failure that the feeling of relief was over-powering. In fact it intoxicated me, so that for a long time I just sailed along, grinning foolishly to myself.

When I finally came to my senses I looked down happily over the side. It must be time to turn now, but as I stared downwards cold reality began to roll over me in a gathering flood. I couldn't recognize a thing in the great hazy tapestry beneath me. And everything seemed smaller than usual. Dry-mouthed, I looked at the altimeter. I was well over two thousand feet.

And suddenly it came to me that FO Woodham's shouts had not been meaningless; he had been talking sense, giving me good advice, and as soon as I got up in the air by myself I had ignored it all. I hadn't lined myself up on a cloud, I hadn't watched my artificial horizon. I hadn't kept an eye on the altimeter. And I was lost.

It was a terrible feeling, this sense of utter isolation as I desperately scanned the great chequered landscape for a familiar object. What did you do in a case like this? Soar around southern England till I found some farmer's field big enough to land in, then make my own abject way back to Winkfield? But that way I was going to look the complete fool, and also I'd stand an excellent chance of smashing up that fitter's beloved aeroplane and maybe myself.

It seemed to me that one way or another I was going to make a name for myself. Funny things had happened to some of the other lads – many had been air-sick and vomited in the cockpit, one had gone through a hedge, another on his first solo had circled the airfield again and again – seven times he had gone round – trying to find the courage to land while his instructor sweated blood and cursed on the ground. But nobody had really got lost like me. Nobody had flown off into the blue and returned on foot without his aeroplane.

My visions of my immediate fate were reaching horrific proportions and my heart was hammering uncontrollably when far away on my left I spotted the dear familiar bulk of the big stand on Ascot racecourse. Almost weeping with joy, I turned towards it and within minutes I was banking above its roof as I had done so often.

And there, far below and approaching with uncomfortable speed was the belt of trees which fringed the airfield, and beyond the windsock blowing over the wide green. But I was still far too high – I could never drop down there in time to hit that landing strip, I would have to go round again.

The ignominy of it went deep. They would all be watching on the ground and some would have a good laugh at the sight of Herriot over-shooting the field by several hundred feet and cruising off again into the clouds. But what was I thinking about?

There was a way of losing height rapidly and, bless you FO Woodham, I knew how to do it.

Opposite rudder and stick. He had told me a hundred times how to side slip and I did it now as hard as I could, sending the little machine slewing like an airborne crab down, down towards those trees.

And by golly it worked! The green copse rushed up at me and before I knew I was almost skimming the branches. I straightened up and headed for the long stretch of grass. At fifty feet I rounded out, then checked the stick gradually back till just above the ground, when I slammed it into my abdomen. The undercarriage made contact with the earth with hardly a tremor and I worked the rudder bar to keep straight until I came to a halt. Then I taxied in, climbed from the cockpit and walked over to the flight hut.

FO Woodham was sitting at a table, cup in hand, and he looked up as I entered. He had got out of his flying suit and was wearing a battle dress jacket with the wings we all dreamed about and the ribbon of the DFC.

'Ah, Herriot, I'm just having some coffee. Will you join me?'

'Thank you, sir.'

I sat down and he pushed a cup towards me.

'I saw your landing,' he said. 'Delightful, quite delightful.'

'Thank you, sir.'

'And that sideslip.' One corner of his mouth twitched upwards. 'Very good indeed, really masterly.'

He reached for the coffee pot and went on. 'You've done awfully well, Herriot. Solo after nine hours' instruction, eh? Splendid. But then I never had the slightest doubt about you at any time.'

He poised the pot over my cup. 'How do you like your coffee — black or white?'

11

I was only the third man in our Flight of fifty to go solo and it was a matter of particular pride to me because so many of my comrades were eighteen- and nineteen-year-olds. They didn't say so but I often had the impression that they felt that an elderly gentleman like me in my twenties with a wife and baby had no right to be there, training for aircrew. In the nicest possible way they thought I was past it.

Of course, in many ways they had a point. The pull I had from home was probably stronger than theirs. When our sergeant handed out the letters on the daily parade I used to secrete mine away till I had a few minutes of solitude to read about how fast little Jimmy was growing, how much he weighed, the unmistakable signs of outstanding intelligence, even genius, which Helen could already discern in him.

I was missing his babyhood and it saddened me. It is still something I deeply regret because it comes only once and is gone so quickly. But I still have the bundles of letters which his proud mother wrote to keep me in touch with every fascinating stage, and when I read them now it is almost as though I had been there to see it all.

At the time, those letters pulled me back almost painfully to the comforts of home but on the other hand there were occasions when life in Darrowby hadn't been all that comfortable . . .

I think it was the early morning calls in the winter which were the worst. It was a fairly common experience to be walking sleepy-eyed into a cow byre at 6 a.m. for a calving, but at Mr Blackburn's farm there was a difference. In fact, several differences.

Firstly, there was usually an anxious-faced farmer to greet me with news of how the calf was coming, when labour had started, but today I was like an unwelcome stranger. Secondly, I had grown accustomed to the sight of a few cows tied up in a cobbled byre with wooden partitions and an oil lamp, and now I was gazing down a long avenue of concrete under blazing electric light with a seemingly endless succession of bovine backsides protruding from tubular metal standings. Thirdly, instead of the early morning peace there was a clattering of buckets, the rhythmic pulsing of a milking machine and the blaring of a radio loud-speaker. There was also a frantic scurrying of white-coated, white-capped men, but none of them paid the slightest attention to me.

This was one of the new big dairy farms. In place of a solitary figure on a milk stool, head buried in the cow's side, pulling forth the milk with a gentle 'hiss-hiss' there was this impersonal hustle and bustle.

I stood just inside the doorway while out in the yard a particularly cold snow drifted from the blackness above. I had left a comfortable bed and a warm wife to come here and it seemed somebody ought at least to say 'hello'. Then I noticed the owner hurrying past with a bucket. He was moving as fast as any of his men.

'Hey, Mr Blackburn!' I cried. 'You rang me – you've got a cow calving?'

He stopped and looked at me uncomprehendingly for a moment. 'Oh aye . . . aye . . . she's down there on t'right.' He pointed to a light roan animal halfway along the byre. She was easy to pick out – the only one lying down.

'How long has she been on?' I asked, but when I turned round Mr Blackburn had gone. I trotted after him, cornered him in the milk house and repeated my question.

'Oh, she should've calved last night. Must be summat amiss.' He began to pour his bucket of milk over the cooler into the churn.

'Have you had a feel inside her?'

'Nay, haven't had time.' He turned harassed eyes towards me. 'We're a bit behind with milkin' this mornin'. We can't be late for t'milk man.'

I knew what he meant. The drivers who collected the churns for the big dairy companies were a fierce body of men. Probably kind husbands and fathers at normal times but subject to violent outbursts of rage if they were kept waiting even for an instant. I couldn't blame them, because they had a lot of territory to cover and many farms to visit, but I had seen them when provoked and their anger was frightening to behold.

'All right,' I said. 'Can I have some hot water, soap and a towel, please?'

103

Mr Blackburn jerked his head at the corner of the milk house. 'You'll 'ave to help yourself. There's everythin' there. Ah must get on.' He went off again at a brisk walk. Clearly he was more in fear of the milk man than he was of me.

I filled a bucket, found a piece of soap and threw a towel over my shoulder. When I reached my patient I looked in vain for some sign of a name. So many of the cows of those days had their names printed above their stalls but there were no Marigolds, Alices or Snowdrops here, just numbers.

Before taking off my jacket I looked casually in the ear where the tattoo marks stood out plainly against the creamy white surface. She was number eighty-seven.

I was in more trouble when I stripped off my shirt. In a modern byre like this there were no nails jutting from the walls to serve as hangers. I had to roll my clothes into a ball and carry them through to the milk house. There I found a sack which I tied round my middle with a length of binder twine.

Still ignored by everybody, I returned, soaped my arm and inserted it into the cow. I had to go a long way in to reach the calf, which was strange considering the birth should have taken place last night. It was the top of the little creature's head I touched first; the nose was tucked downwards instead of thrusting its way along the vagina towards the outside world, and the legs were similarly coiled under the body.

And I noticed something else. The entry of my arm did not provoke any answering strain from the cow, nor did she try to rise to her feet. There was something else troubling Number Eighty-Seven.

Lying flat on the concrete, still buried to the shoulder in the cow, I raised my head and looked along the shaggy back with its speckle of light red and white hairs, and when I reached the neck I knew I need seek no further. The lateral kink was very obvious. Number Eighty-Seven, slumped on her chest, was gazing wearily and without interest at the wall in front of her but there was that funny little bend in her neck that told me everything.

I got up, washed and dried my arm and looked for Mr Blackburn. I found him bending by the side of a fat brown animal, pulling the cups from her teats. I tapped him on the shoulder.

'She's got milk fever.' I said.

'Oh, aye,' he replied, then he hoisted the bucket, brushed past me and made off down the byre.

I kept pace with him. 'That's why she can't strain. Her uterus has lost its tone. She'll never calve till she gets some calcium.'

'Right.' He still didn't look at me. 'Ye'll give 'er some, then?'

'Yes,' I said to his retreating back.

The snow still swirled in the outer darkness and I toyed with the idea of getting dressed. But I'd only have to strip again so I decided to make a dash for it. With the car boot open, it seemed to take a long time to fish out the bottles and flutter valve with the flakes settling thickly on my naked flesh.

Back in the byre I looked around for a spare man to help me but there was no lessening of the feverish activity. I would have to roll this cow on to her side and inject into her milk vein without assistance. It all depended on how comatose she was.

And she must have been pretty far gone because when I braced my feet against the tubular steel and pushed both hands against her shoulder she flopped over without resistance. To keep her there I lay on top of her as I pushed in the needle and ran the calcium into the vein.

One snag was that my sprawling position took me right underneath the neighbouring cow on the right, a skittish sort of animal who didn't welcome the rubber-booted legs tangling with her hind feet. She expressed her disapproval by treading painfully on my ankles and giving me a few smart kicks on the thigh, but I dared not move because the calcium was flowing in beautifully.

When the bottle was empty I kneed my patient back on to her chest and ran another bottle of calcium magnesium and phosphorus under her skin. By the time I had finished and rubbed away the subcutaneous fluid Number Eighty-Seven was looking decidedly happier.

I didn't hurry over cleaning and putting away my injection outfit and re-soaping my arms because I knew that every minute would bring back strength to my patient.

The lightning response to intravenous calcium has always afforded me a simple pleasure and when I pushed my arm in again the difference was remarkable. The previously flaccid uterus gripped at my hand and as the cow went into a long expulsive effort she turned her head, looked back at me and opened her mouth in a muffled bellow. It was not a sound of pain but rather as though she was saying, 'I'm back in business now.'

'All right, my lass,' I replied. 'I'll stay with you till it's all over.'

At other times I might have been a little chary of being over-heard conversing with a cow, but with the clamour of buckets and the nonstop blasting of the radio there was no chance of that happening.

I knew that I had to guide the calf back into the correct position and that it would take time, but I had a strange sense of one-ness with this animal because neither of us seemed to be of the slightest importance in the present setting. As I lay there face down on the concrete which grew harder all the time and with the milkers stumbling over my prostrate form I felt very much alone. There was just myself and Number Eighty-Seven for it.

Another thing I missed was the sense of occasion. There was a compensation in many an arduous calving in the feeling of a little drama being enacted; the worried farmer, attentive stockmen, the danger of losing the calf or even the mother – it was a gripping play and there was no doubt the vet was the leading man. He may even be the villain but he was number one. And here I was now, a scrabbling nonentity with hardly a mention in the cast. It was the shape of things to come.

And yet . . . and yet . . . the job was still there. I lifted the calf's lower jaw and as the cow gave a heave I eased it over the brim of the pelvis. Then I groped for the tiny legs and straightened them as another expulsive effort pushed the little creature towards me. He was definitely on his way now.

I didn't rush things – just lay there and let the cow get on with it. My worst moment was when one of the men came to put the milking machine on the temperamental animal on my right. As he tried to step up beside her she swung round, cocked her tail and sent a jet of faeces cascading across my back.

The man pushed her back into place, slipped on the teat cups then lifted the hose which was lying ready for swilling down the byre. A moment later I felt the icy flow of water playing from my shoulders to my hips, then the application of a spare udder cloth as the helpful fellow cleaned me off.

'Thanks very much,' I gasped. And I was really grateful. It was the only attention I had received all morning.

Within half an hour the feet appeared at the vulva followed by a wet nose whose nostrils twitched reassuringly. But they were big feet – this would be a bull calf and his final entry into the world could be a tight squeeze.

I got into a sitting position and gripped a slippery cloven hoof in each hand. Leaning back, feet against the dung channel, I addressed Number Eighty-Seven again.

'Come on, old lass. A couple of good shoves and we're there.'

She responded with a mighty inflation of the abdomen and the calf surged towards me as I pulled, giving me a glimpse of a broad forehead and a pair of slightly puzzled eyes. For a moment I thought the ears were going to slip through but then the cow relaxed and the head disappeared back inside.

'Once more, girl!' I pleaded, and this time it seemed that she had decided to stop playing around and get the job over with. She gave a prolonged strain which sent head and shoulders through, and as I hauled away I had only that momentary panic I always feel that the hips might jam in the pelvis. But this one didn't stick and came sliding beautifully on to my lap.

Puffing slightly, I got to my feet and parted the hind legs. Sure enough the little scrotum was there; he was a fine bull calf. I pulled some hay from the rack and dried him off and within minutes he was sitting up, sniffing and snorting, looking around him with interest.

He wasn't the only interested party. His mother, craning round in her neck chain, gazed fascinatedly at the new arrival before releasing a deafening bellow. I seized the front feet again and pulled the calf up to the front of the stall where the cow, after a brief examination, began to lick him from head to tail. Then as I watched, entranced, she suddenly rose to her feet so that she could reach some of the little creature's more inaccessible corners.

I smiled to myself. So that was that. She had got over the milk fever and had a nice live calf, too. All was well with Number Eighty-Seven.

Mr Blackburn came up and stood by my side and I realized that the noise in the byre had subsided. The milking was finished.

The farmer took off his white hat and wiped away the sweat

from his brow. 'By gaw, that was a rush. We were short-handed this mornin' and I was sure we were goin' to miss that milk feller. He's a terror – won't wait a minute, and I've had to chase after 'im in a tractor with the churns afore now.'

As he finished speaking a hen leaped with a squawk from the rack. Mr Blackburn reached forward and lifted a warm new-laid egg out of the hay.

He inspected it for a moment then turned to me. 'Have you 'ad your breakfast ?'

'No, of course not.'

'Well, tell your missus to put this in the fryin' pan,' he said, handing me the egg.

'Oh, thank you very much, Mr Blackburn, I'll enjoy that.'

He nodded and continued to stand there, gazing at the cow and calf. Dairy farming is one of the hardest ways of making a living and this pre-dawn turmoil was an everyday occurrence in his life. But I knew he was pleased with my efforts because he faced me suddenly and his weathered features broke into a delighted grin. Without warning he gave me a friendly thump on the chest.

'Good old Jim!' he said, and walked away.

I dressed, got into the car and placed my egg with the utmost care on the dash, then I eased myself gingerly on to the seat, because that hosing had sent a pint or two of dirty water down into my underpants and sitting down was intensely uncomfortable.

As I drove away the darkness was thinning into the grey beginning of a new day and around me the white bulk of the fells began to lift from the half light – massive, smooth and inexpressibly cold.

I looked at the egg rocking gently on the dash, and smiled to myself. I could still see Mr Blackburn's sudden grin, still feel his punch on the chest, and my main sensation was of reassurance.

Systems may be changing, but cows and calves and Yorkshire farmers were just the same.

12

On my wage of seven and threepence a day, out of which was deducted maintenance for wife and child, I was unable to indulge in high living even if I had wanted to, but one evening in Windsor I decided to allow myself the luxury of one glass of beer, and as I pushed open the pub doorway the first thing I saw was a man sitting at the corner of the bar with a small dog under his chair.

Little things like that could lift me effortlessly back to my old life, and I could almost hear George Wilks, the auctioneer, in the Drovers' Arms at Darrowby.

'I reckon that's the best pub terrier I've ever seen.' He bent down from the bar counter and patted Theo's shaggy head as it protruded from beneath his master's stool.

It struck me that 'pub terrier' wasn't a bad description. Theo was small and mainly white, though there were odd streaks of black on his flanks, and his muzzle had a bushy outgrowth of hair which made him undeniably attractive but still more mysterious.

I warmed to a Scottish colleague recently who, when pressed by a lady client to diagnose her dog's breed and lineage replied finally, 'Madam, I think it would be best just to call him a wee broon dug.'

By the same token Theo could be safely be described as a wee white dug, but in Yorkshire the expression 'pub terrier' would be more easily understood.

His master, Paul Cotterell, looked down from his high perch. 'What's he saying about you, old chap ?' he murmured languidly, and at the sound of his voice the little animal leaped, eager and wagging, from his retreat.

Theo spent a considerable part of his life between the four metal legs of that stool, as did his master on the seat. And it often seemed to me to be a waste of time for both of them. I often took my own dog, Sam, into pubs and he could squat beneath my seat, but whereas it was an occasional thing with me – maybe once or twice a week – with Paul Cotterell it was an unvarying ritual. Every night from eight o'clock onwards he could be found sitting there at the end of the bar of the Drovers' Arms, pint glass in front of him, little curly pipe drooping over his chin.

For a young man like him – he was a bachelor in his late thirties – and a person of education and intelligence, it seemed a sterile existence.

He turned to me as I approached the counter. 'Hello, Jim, let me get you a drink.'

'That's very kind of you, Paul,' I replied. 'I'll have a pint.'

'Splendid.' He turned to the barmaid with easy courtesy. 'Could I trouble you, Moyra ?'

We sipped our beer and we chatted. This time it was about the music festival at Brawton and then we got on to music in general. As with any other topic I had discussed with him he seemed to know a lot about it.

'So you're not all that keen on Bach ?' he inquired lazily.

'No, not really. Some of it, yes, but on the whole I like something a bit more emotional. Elgar, Beethoven, Mozart. Even Tchaikovsky – I suppose you highbrows look down your noses at him ?'

He shrugged, puffed his little pipe and regarded me with a half-smile, one eyebrow raised. He often looked like that and it made me feel he ought to wear a monocle. But he didn't enthuse about Bach, though it seemed he was his favourite composer. He never enthused about anything, and he listened with that funny look on his face while I rhapsodized about the Elgar violin concerto.

Paul Cotterell was from the south of England, but the locals had long since forgiven him for that because he was likeable, amusing, and always ready to buy anybody a drink from his corner in the Drovers'. To me, he had a charm which was very English; casual, effortless. He never got excited, he was always polite and utterly self-contained.

'While you're here, Jim,' he said. 'I wonder if you'd have a look at Theo's foot ?'

'Of course.' It is one of a vet's occupational hazards that wherever he goes socially it is taken for granted that there is nothing he would rather do than dole out advice or listen to symptoms. 'Let's have him up.'

'Here, boy, come on.' Paul patted his knee and the little dog jumped up and sat there, eyes sparkling with pleasure. And I thought as I always did that Theo should be in pictures. He was the perfect film dog with that extraordinarily fuzzy laugh-face. People paid good money to see dogs just like him in cinemas all over the world.

'All right, Theo,' I said, scooping him from his master's knee. 'Where's the trouble?'

Paul indicated the right forefoot with the stem of his pipe. 'It's that one. He's been going a bit lame off and on for the last few days.'

'I see.' I rolled the little animal on his back and then laughed. 'Oh, he's only got a broken claw. There's a little bit hanging off here. He must have caught it on a stone. Hang on a minute.' I delved in my pocket for the scissors which always dwelt there. A quick snip and the job was done.

'Is that all?' asked Paul.

'Yes, that's it.'

One eyebrow went up mockingly as he looked at Theo. 'So that's what you were making all the fuss about, eh? Silly old trout.' He snapped his fingers. 'Back you go.'

The little dog obediently leaped to the carpet and disappeared into his sanctuary beneath the stool. And at that moment I had a flash of intuition about Paul – about his charm which I had often admired and envied. He didn't really care. He was fond of his dog, of course. He took him everywhere with him, exercised him regularly by the river, but there was none of the anxiety, the almost desperate concern which I had so often seen in the eyes of my clients when I dealt with even the most trivial of their ailments. They cared too much – as I have always done with my own animals.

And of course he was right. It was an easier and more comfortable way to live. Caring made you vulnerable, while Paul cruised along, impregnable. That attractive casualness, the nonchalant good manners, the imperturbability – they all had their roots in the fact that nothing touched him very deeply.

And despite my snap diagnosis of his character I still envied him. I have always been blown around too easily by my emotions; it must be lovely to be like Paul. And the more I thought about it the more I realized how everything fitted in. He had

111

never cared enough to get married. Even Bach, with his mathematical music, was part of the pattern.

'I think that major operation deserves another pint, Jim.' He smiled his lop-sided smile. 'Unless you demand a higher fee?'

I laughed. I would always like him. We are all different and we have to act as we are made, but as I started my second glass I thought again of his carefree life. He had a good job in the government offices in Brawton, no domestic responsibilities, and every night he sat on that same stool drinking beer with his dog underneath. He hadn't a worry in the world.

Anyway, he was part of the Darrowby scene, part of something I liked, and since I have always hated change it was in a sense reassuring to know that no matter what night you went into the Drovers' you would find Paul Cotterell in the corner and Theo's shaggy muzzle peeping from below.

I felt like that one night when I dropped in near closing time.

'D'you think he's got worms?' The question was typically off-hand.

'I don't know, Paul. Why do you ask?'

He drew on his pipe. 'Oh, I just thought he looked a bit thin lately. Come up, Theo!'

The little dog, perched on his master's knee, looked as chirpy as ever and when I reached over and lifted him he licked my hand. But his ribs did feel rather prominent.

'Mmm, yes,' I said. 'Maybe he has lost a bit of weight. Have you noticed him passing any worms?'

'I haven't, actually.'

'Not even little bits – whitish segments sticking round his rear?'

'No, Jim.' He shook his head and smiled. 'But I haven't looked all that closely, old boy.'

'Okay,' I said. 'Let's worm him, just in case. I'll bring in some tablets tomorrow night. You'll be here ...?'

The eyebrow went up. 'I think that's highly probable.'

Theo duly got his worm tablets and after that there was a space of several weeks when I was too busy to visit the Drovers'. When I finally did get in it was a Saturday night and the Athletic Club dance was in full spate. A rhythmic beat drifted from the ball-room, the little bar was packed, and the domino players were under pressure, squashed into a corner by the crush of dinner jackets and backless dresses.

In the noise and heat I struggled towards the bar, thinking that the place was unrecognizable. But there was one feature unchanged – Paul Cotterell on his stool at the far end of the counter.

I squeezed in next to him and saw he was wearing his usual tweed jacket. 'Not dancing, Paul?'

He half closed his eyes, shook his head slowly and smiled at me over his bent little pipe. 'Not for me, old boy,' he murmured. 'Too much like work.'

I glanced down and saw that something else hadn't changed. Theo was there, too, keeping his nose well clear of the milling feet. I ordered two beers and we tried to converse, but it was difficult to shout above the babel. Arms kept poking between us towards the counter, red faces pushed into ours and shouted greetings. Most of the time we just looked around us.

Then Paul leaned close and spoke into my ear. 'I gave Theo those pills but he's still getting thinner.'

'Really?' I shouted back. 'That's unusual.'

'Yes . . . perhaps you'd have a look at him?'

I nodded, he snapped his fingers and the little dog was on his knee in an instant. I reached and lifted him on to mine and I noticed immediately that he was lighter in my hands.

'You're right,' I said. 'He's still losing weight.'

Balancing the dog in my lap, I pulled down an eyelid and saw that the conjunctiva was pale.

I shouted again. 'He's anaemic.' I felt my way back over his face and behind the angle of the jaw I found that the post-pharyngeal lymph glands were greatly enlarged. This was strange. Could he have some form of mouth or throat infection? I looked helplessly around me, wishing fervently that Paul wouldn't invariably consult me about his dog in a pub. I wanted to examine the animal, but I couldn't very well deposit him among the glasses on the bar.

I was trying to get a better grip with a view to looking down his throat when my hand slipped behind his foreleg and my heart gave a sudden thump as I encountered the axillary gland. It, too, was grossly enlarged. I whipped my fingers back into his groin and there was the inguinal gland, prominent as an egg. The pre-scapular was the same, and as I groped feverishly I realized that every superficial lymph gland was several times its normal size.

Hodgkin's disease. For a few moments I was oblivious of the shouting and laughter, the muffled blare of music. Then I looked at Paul who was regarding me calmly as he puffed his pipe. How could I tell him in these surroundings ? He would ask me what Hodgkin's disease was and I would have to explain that it was a cancer of the lymphatic system and that his dog was surely going to die.

As my thoughts raced I stroked the shaggy head and Theo's comic whiskered face turned towards me. People jostled past, hands reached out and bore gins and whiskies and beers past my face, a fat man threw his arm round my neck.

I leaned across. 'Paul,' I said.

'Yes, Jim ?'

'Will you . . . will you bring Theo round to the surgery to-morrow morning. It's ten o'clock on a Sunday.'

Momentarily the eyebrow twitched upwards, then he nodded. 'Right, old boy.'

I didn't bother to finish my drink. I began to push my way towards the door and as the crush closed around me I glanced back. The little dog's tail was just disappearing under the stool.

Next day I had one of those early waking mornings when I started tossing around at six o'clock and finished by staring at the ceiling.

Even after I had got my feet on the ground and brought Helen a cup of tea, the waiting was interminable until the moment arrived which I had been dreading – when I faced Paul across the surgery table with Theo standing between us.

I told him straight away. I couldn't think of any easy way to lead up to it.

His expression did not change, but he took his pipe out of his mouth and looked steadily at me, then at the dog and back again at me.

'Oh,' he said at last. 'I see.'

I didn't say anything and he slowly ran his hand along the little animal's back. 'Are you quite sure, Jim ?'

'Absolutely. I'm terribly sorry.'

'Is there no treatment ?'

'There are various palliatives, Paul, but I've never seen any of them do any good. The end result is always the same.'

'Yes . . .' He nodded slowly. 'But he doesn't look so bad. What will happen if we don't do anything ?'

I paused. 'Well, as the internal glands enlarge, various things will happen. Ascites – dropsy – will develop in the abdomen. In fact you see he's a little bit pot-bellied now.'

'Yes . . . I do see, now you mention it. Anything else ?'

'As the thoracic glands get bigger he'll begin to pant.'

'I've noticed that already. He's breathless after a short walk.'

'And all the time he'll get thinner and thinner and more debilitated.'

Paul looked down at his feet for a few moments then faced me. 'So what it amounts to is that he's going to be pretty miserable for the rest of his life.' He swallowed. 'And how long is that going to be ?'

'A few weeks. It varies. Maybe up to three months.'

'Well, Jim.' He smoothed back his hair. 'I can't let that happen. It's my responsibility. You must put him to sleep now, before he really starts to suffer. Don't you agree ?'

'Yes, Paul, it's the kindest thing to do.'

'Will you do it immediately – as soon as I am out of that door ?'

'I will,' I replied. 'And I promise you he won't know a thing.'

His face held a curious fixity of expression. He put his pipe in his mouth, but it had gone out so he stuffed it into his pocket. Then he leaned forward and patted his dog once on the head. The bushy face with the funny shock of hair round the muzzle turned to him and for a few seconds they looked at each other.

Then, 'Goodbye, old chap,' he muttered and strode quickly from the room.

I kept my promise.

'Good lad, good old Theo,' I murmured, and stroked the face and ears again and again as the little creature slipped peacefully away. Like all vets I hated doing this, painless though it was, but to me there has always been a comfort in the knowledge that the last thing these helpless animals knew was the sound of a friendly voice and the touch of a gentle hand.

Sentimental, maybe. Not like Paul. He had been practical and utterly rational in the way he had acted. He had been able to do the right thing because he was not at the mercy of his emotions.

Later, over a Sunday lunch which I didn't enjoy as much as usual I told Helen about Theo.

I had to say something because she had produced a delicious pot roast on the gas ring which was our only means of cooking and I wasn't doing justice to her skill.

Sitting at our bench I looked down at her. It was my turn for the high stool.

'You know, Helen,' I said, 'that was an object lesson for me. The way Paul acted, I mean. If I'd been in his position I'd have shilly-shallied – tried to put off something which was inevitable.'

She thought for a moment. 'Well, a lot of people would.'

'Yes, but he didn't.' I put down my knife and fork and stared at the wall. 'He behaved in a mature way. I suppose Paul has one of those personalities you read about. Well-adjusted, completely adequate.'

'Come on, Jim, eat your lunch. I know it was a sad thing but it had to be done and you mustn't start criticizing yourself. Paul is Paul and you are you.'

I started again on the meat but I couldn't repress the rising sense of my own inadequacy. Then as I glanced to one side I saw that my wife was smiling up at me.

I felt suddenly reassured. It seemed that she at least didn't seem to mind that I was me.

That was on the Sunday, and on Tuesday morning I was handing out some wart lotion to Mr Sangster who kept a few dairy cows down by the station.

'Dab that on the udder night and morning after milking,' I said. 'I think you'll find that the warts will start to drop off after a week or two.'

'Thank ye.' He handed over half a crown and I was dropping it into the desk drawer when he spoke again.

'Bad job about Paul Cotterell, wasn't it?'

'What do you mean?'

'Ah thought you'd have heard,' he said. 'He's dead.'

'Dead!' I stared at him stupidly. 'How ... what ... ?'

'Found 'im this mornin'. He did away with 'isself.'

I leaned with both hands on the desk. 'Do you mean . . . suicide?'

'Aye, that's what they say. Took a lot o' pills. It's all ower t'town.'

I found myself hunching over the day book, sightlessly scanning the list of calls while the farmer's voice seemed to come from far away.

'It's a bad job, right enough. He were a nice feller. Reckon everybody liked 'im.'

Later that day I was passing Paul's lodgings when I saw his landlady, Mrs Clayton, in the doorway. I pulled up and got out of the car.

'Mrs Clayton,' I said. 'I still can't believe this.'

'Nor can I, Mr Herriot, it's terrible.' Her face was pale, her eyes red. 'He was with me six years, you know – he was like a son.'

'But why on earth . . . ?'

'Oh, it was losin' his dog that did it. He just couldn't stand it.'

A great wave of misery rose and engulfed me and she put her hand on my arm.

'Don't look like that, Mr Herriot. It wasn't your fault. Paul told me all about it and nobody could have saved Theo. People die of that, never mind dogs.'

I nodded dumbly and she went on.

'But I'll tell your something in confidence, Mr Herriot. Paul wasn't able to stand things like you or me. It was the way he was made – you see he suffered from depression.'

'Depression! Paul . . . ?'

'Oh yes, he's been under the doctor for a long time and takin' pills regular. He allus put a brave face on, but he's had nervous trouble off and on for years.'

'Nervous trouble . . . I'd never have dreamed . . .'

'No, nobody would, but that's how it was. He had an unhappy childhood from what I made out. Maybe that's why he was so fond of his dog. He got too attached to him, really.'

'Yes . . . yes . . .'

She took out a screwed up handkerchief and blew her nose. 'Well, as I said, the poor lad had a rough time most of his life, but he was brave.'

There didn't seem anything else to say. I drove away out of the town and the calm green hills offered a quiet contrast to the turmoil which can fill a man's mind. So much for Herriot as a judge of character. I couldn't have been more wrong, but Paul had fought his secret battle with a courage which had deceived everybody.

I reflected on the object lesson which I thought he had given me, but in fact it was a lesson of another kind and one which I have never forgotten; that there are countless people like Paul who are not what they seem.

13

The shock of Paul Cotterell's death stayed with me for a long time, and in fact I know I have never quite got over it because even now when the company in the bar of the Drovers' has changed and I am one of the few old faces left from thirty-five years ago I can still see the jaunty figure on the corner stool and the bushy face peeping from beneath.

It was the kind of experience I didn't want repeated in my lifetime yet, uncannily, I ran into the same sort of thing almost immediately afterwards.

It couldn't have been more than a week after Paul's funeral that Andrew Vine brought his fox terrier to the surgery.

I put the little dog on the table and examined each of his eyes carefully in turn.

'I'm afraid he's getting worse,' I said.

Without warning the man slumped across the table and buried his face in his hands.

I put my hand on his shoulder. 'What is it, Andrew? What on earth's the matter?'

At first he did not answer but stayed there, huddled grotesquely by the side of his dog as great sobs shook his body.

When he spoke at last it was into his hands and his voice was hoarse and desperate. 'I can't stand it! If Digger goes blind I'll kill myself!'

I looked down at the bowed head in horrified disbelief. It couldn't be happening again. Not so soon after Paul. And yet there were similarities. Andrew was another bachelor in his thirties and the terrier was his constant companion. He lived in lodgings and appeared to have no worries though he was a shy, diffident man with a fragile look about his tall stooping frame and pallid face.

He had first consulted me about Digger several months ago.

'I call him that because he's dug large holes in the garden ever since his puppy days,' he said with a half-smile, looking at me almost apprehensively from large dark eyes.

I laughed. 'I hope you haven't brought him to me to cure that, because I've never read anything in the books about it.'

'No, no, it's about something else – his eyes. And he's had that trouble since he was a pup, too.'

'Really? Tell me.'

'Well, when I first got him he had sort of mattery eyes, but the breeder said he'd probably just got some irritant in them and it would soon clear up. And in fact it did. But he's never been quite right. He always seems to have a little discomfort in his eyes.'

'How do you mean?'

'He rubs the side of his face along the carpet and he blinks in bright light.'

'I see.' I pulled the little animal's face round towards me and looked intently at the eyelids. My mind had been busy as he spoke and I was fairly sure I should find either entropion (inversion of the eyelids) or distichiasis (an extra row of lashes rubbing against the eyeball), but there was no sign of either. The surface of the cornea, too, looked normal, except perhaps that the deeper structure of lens and iris were not as easy to define as usual.

I moved over to a cupboard for the ophthalmoscope. 'How old is he now?'

'About a year.'

'So he's had this for about ten months?'

'Yes, about that. But it varies a lot. Most of the time he seems normal, then there are days when he goes and lies in his basket with his eyes half closed and you can tell there's something wrong. Not pain, really. More like discomfort, as I said.'

I nodded and hoped I was looking wise but none of this added up to anything familiar. I switched on the little light on the ophthalmoscope and peered into the depths of that most magical and delicate of all organs, down through the lens to the brilliant tapestry of the retina with its optic papilla and branching blood vessels. I couldn't find a thing wrong.

'Does he still dig holes?' I asked. When baffled I often snatch at straws and I wondered if the dog was suffering from a soil irritation.

Andrew shook his head. 'No, very seldom now, and anyway, his bad days are never associated with his digging.'

'Is that so?' I rubbed my chin. The man was obviously ahead of me with his thinking and I had an uncomfortable feeling of bewilderment. People were always bringing their dogs in with 'bad eyes' and there was invariably something to be seen, some cause to be found. 'And would you say that this was one of his bad days?'

'Well I thought so this morning, but he seems a bit better now. Still, he's a bit blinky, don't you think?'

'Yes . . . maybe so.' Digger did appear to be reluctant to open his eyes fully to the sunshine streaming through the surgery window. And occasionally he kept them closed for a second or two as though he wasn't very happy. But damn it, nothing gave me the slightest clue.

I didn't tell the owner that I hadn't the faintest idea what was wrong with his dog. Such remarks do not inspire confidence. Instead, I took refuge in businesslike activity.

'I'm going to give you some lotion,' I said briskly. 'Put a few drops into his eyes three times daily. And let me know how he goes on. It's possible he has some long-standing infection in there.'

I handed over a bottle of two per cent boric acid solution and patted Digger's head. 'I hope that will clear things up for you, lad,' I said, and the stumpy tail wagged in reply. He was a sharp looking little animal, attractive and good-natured and a fine specimen of the smooth-haired breed with his long head and neck, pointed nose and beautifully straight limbs.

He jumped from the table and leaped excitedly around his master's legs.

I laughed. 'He's eager to go, like most of my patients.' I bent and slapped him playfully on the rump. 'My word, doesn't he look fit!'

'He is fit.' Andrew smiled proudly. 'In fact I often think that apart from those eyes he's a perfect little physical machine. You should see him out in the fields – he can run like a whippet.'

'I'll bet he can. Keep in touch, will you?' I waved them out of the door and turned to my other work, mercifully unaware that I had just embarked on one of the most frustrating and traumatic cases of my career.

After that first time I took special notice of Digger and his owner. Andrew, a sensitive likeable man, was a representative for a firm of agricultural chemists and, like myself, spent most of his time driving around the Darrowby district. His dog was always with him and I had been perfunctorily amused by the fact that the little animal was invariably peering intently through the windscreen, his paws either on the dash or balanced on his master's hand as he operated the gear lever.

But now that I was personally interested I could discern the obvious delight which the little animal derived from taking in every detail of his surroundings. He missed nothing in his daily journeys. The road ahead, the houses and people, trees and fields which flashed by the windows – these made up his world.

I met him one day when I was exercising Sam up on the high moors which crown the windy summits of the fells. But this was May, the air was soft and a week's hot sunshine had dried the green paths which wandered among the heather. I saw Digger flashing like a white streak over the velvet turf and when he spotted Sam he darted up to him, set himself teasingly for a moment, then shot back to Andrew who was standing in a natural circular glade among the harsh brown growth.

Here gorse bushes blazed in full yellow glory and the little dog hurtled round and round the arena, exulting in his health and speed.

'That's what I'd call sheer joy of living,' I said.

Andrew smiled shyly. 'Yes, isn't he beautiful,' he murmured.

'How are the eyes?' I asked.

He shrugged. 'Sometimes good, sometimes not so good. Much the same as before. But I must say he seems easier whenever I put the drops in.'

'But he still has days when he looks unhappy?'

'Yes ... I have to say yes. Some days they bother him a lot.'

Again the frustration welled in me. 'Let's walk back to the car,' I said. 'I might as well have a look at him.'

I lifted Digger on to the bonnet and examined him again. There wasn't a single abnormality in the eyelids – I had wondered if I had missed something last time – but as the bright sunshine slanted across the eyeballs I could just discern the faintest cloudiness in the cornea. There was a slight keratitis there which hadn't been visible before. But why ... why?

'He'd better have some stronger lotion.' I rummaged in the car boot. 'I've got some here. We'll try silver nitrate this time.'

Andrew brought him in about a week later. The corneal discoloration had gone – probably the silver nitrate had moved it – but the underlying trouble was unchanged. There was still something sadly wrong. Something I couldn't diagnose.

That was when I started to get really worried. As the weeks passed I bombarded those eyes with everything in the book; oxide of mercury, chinosol, zinc sulphide, ichthyol and a host of other things which are now buried in history.

I had none of the modern sophisticated antibiotic and steroid applications but it would have made no difference if I had. I know that now.

The real nightmare started when I saw the first of the pigment cells beginning to invade the cornea. Sinister brown specks gathering at the limbus and pushing out dark tendrils into the smooth membrane which was Digger's window on the world. I had seen cells like them before. When they came they usually stayed. And they were opaque.

Over the next month I fought them with my pathetic remedies, but they crept inwards, slowly but inexorably, blurring and narrowing Digger's field of vision. Andrew noticed them too, and when he brought the little dog into the surgery he clasped and unclasped his hands anxiously.

'You know, he's seeing less all the time, Mr Herriot. I can tell. He still looks out of the car windows but he used to bark at all sorts of things he didn't like – other dogs for instance – and now he just doesn't spot them. He's – he's losing his sight.'

I felt like screaming or kicking the table, but since that wouldn't have helped I just looked at him.

'It's that brown stuff isn't it ?' he said. 'What is it ?'

'It's called pigmentary keratitis, Andrew. It sometimes happens when the cornea – the front of the eyeball – has been inflamed over a long period, and it is very difficult to treat. I'll do the best I can.'

My best wasn't enough. That slow, creeping tide was pitiless, and as the pigment cells were laid down thicker and thicker the resulting layer was almost black, lowering a dingy curtain between Digger and all the things he had gazed at so eagerly.

And all the time I suffered a long gnawing worry, a helpless wretchedness as I contemplated the inevitable.

It was when I examined the eyes five months after I had first seen them that Andrew broke down. There was hardly anything to be seen of the original corneal structure now; just a brown-black opacity which left only minute chinks for moments of sight. Blindness was not far away.

I patted the man's shoulder again. 'Come on, Andrew. Come over here and sit down.' I pulled over the single wooden chair in the consulting room.

He staggered across the floor and almost collapsed on the seat. He sat there, head in hands, for some time then raised a tear-stained face to me. His expression was distraught.

'I can't bear the thought of it,' he gasped. 'A friendly little thing like Digger – he loves everybody. What has he ever done to deserve this ?'

'Nothing, Andrew. It's just one of the sad things which happen. I'm terribly sorry.'

He rolled his head from side to side. 'Oh God, but it's worse for him. You've seen him in the car – he's so interested in everything. Life wouldn't be worth living for him if he lost his sight. And I don't want to live any more either!'

'You mustn't talk like that, Andrew,' I said. 'That's going too far.' I hesitated. 'Please don't be offended, but you ought to see your doctor.'

'Oh, I'm always at the doctor,' he replied dully. 'I'm full of pills right now. He tells me I have a depression.'

The word was like a mournful knell. Coming so soon after Paul it sent a wave of panic through me.

'How long have you been like this ?'

'Oh, weeks. I seem to be getting worse.'

'Have you ever had it before ?'

'No, never.' He wrung his hands and looked at the floor. 'The doctor says that if I keep on taking the pills I'll get over it, but I'm reaching the end of my tether now.'

'But the doctor is right, Andrew. You've got to stick it and you'll be as good as new.'

'I don't believe it,' he muttered. 'Every day lasts a year. I never enjoy anything. And every morning when I wake up I dread having to face the world again.'

I didn't know what to say or how to help. 'Can I get you a glass of water ?'

'No . . . no thanks.'

He turned his deathly pale face up to me again and the dark eyes held a terrible blankness. 'What's the use of going on ? I know I'm going to be miserable for the rest of my life.'

I am no psychiatrist but I knew better than to tell somebody in Andrew's condition to snap out of it. And I had a flash of intuition.

'All right,' I said. 'Be miserable for the rest of your life, but while you're about it you've got to look after this dog.'

'Look after him ? What can I do ? He's going blind. There's nothing anybody can do for him now.'

'You're wrong, Andrew. This is where you start doing things for him. He's going to be lost without your help.'

'How do you mean ?'

'Well, you know all those walks you take him – you've got to get him used to the same tracks and paths so that he can trot along on familiar ground without fear. Keep him clear of holes and ditches.'

He screwed up his face. 'Yes, but he won't enjoy the walks any more.'

'He will,' I said. 'You'll be surprised.'

'Oh, but . . .'

'And that nice big lawn at the back of your house where he runs. You'll have to be on the lookout all the time in case there are things left lying around on the grass that he might bump into. And the eye drops – you say they make him more comfortable. Who's going to put them in if you don't ?'

'But Mr Herriot . . . you've seen how he always looks out of the car when he's with me . . .'

'He'll still look out.'

'Even if he can't see ?'

'Yes.' I put my hand on his arm. 'You must understand, Andrew, when an animal loses his sight he doesn't realize what's happened to him. It's a terrible thing, I know, but he doesn't suffer the mental agony of a human being.'

He stood up and took a long shuddering breath. 'But I'm having the agony. I've been dreading this happening for so long. I haven't been able to sleep for thinking about it. It seems so cruel and unjust for this to strike a helpless animal – a little creature who's never done anybody any harm.' He began to wring his hands again and pace about the room.

'You're just torturing yourself!' I said sharply. 'That's part of your trouble. You're using Digger to punish yourself instead of doing something useful.'

'Oh, but what can I do that will really help ? All those things you talked about – they can't give him a happy life.'

'Oh, but they can. Digger can be happy for years and years if you really work at it. It's up to you.'

Like a man in a dream he bent and gathered his dog into his arms and shuffled along the passage to the front door. As he went down the steps into the street I called out to him.

'Keep in touch with your doctor, Andrew. Take your pills regularly – and remember,' I raised my voice to a shout, 're-member you've got a job to do with that dog!'

*

After Paul, I was on a knife edge of apprehension but this time there was no tragic news to shatter me. Instead I saw Andrew Vine frequently, sometimes in the town with Digger on a lead, occasionally in his car with the little white head framed always in the windscreen, and most often in the fields by the river where he seemed to be carrying out my advice by following the good open tracks again and again.

It was by the river that I stopped him one day. 'How are things going, Andrew ?'

He looked at me unsmilingly. 'Oh, he's finding his way around not too badly. I keep my eye on him. I always avoid that field over there – there's a lot of boggy places in it.'

'Good, that's the idea. And how are you yourself ?'

'Do you really want to know ?'

'Yes, of course.'

He tried to smile. 'Well, this is one of my good days. I'm just tense and dreadfully unhappy. On my bad days I'm terror-stricken, despairing, utterly desolate.'

'I'm sorry, Andrew.'

He shrugged. 'Don't think I'm wallowing in self-pity. You asked me. Anyway, I have a system. Every morning I look at myself in the mirror and I say, 'Okay, Vine, here's another bloody awful day coming up, but you're going to do your job and you're going to look after your dog.'

'That's good, Andrew. And it will all pass. The whole thing will go away and you'll be all right one day.'

'That's what the doctor says.' He gave me a sidelong glance. 'But in the meantime . . .' He looked down at his dog. 'Come on, Digger.'

He turned and strode away abruptly with the little dog trotting after him, and there was something in the set of the man's shoulders and the forward thrust of his head which gave me hope. He was a picture of fierce determination.

My hopes were fulfilled. Both Andrew and Digger won through. I knew that within months, but the final picture in my mind is of a meeting I had with the two of them about two years later. It was on the flat table-land above Darrowby where I had first seen Digger hurtling joyously among the gorse bushes.

He wasn't doing so badly now, running freely over the smooth green turf, sniffing among the herbage, cocking a leg now and then with deep contentment against the drystone wall which ran along the hillside.

Andrew laughed when he saw me. He had put on weight and looked a different person. 'Digger knows every inch of this walk,' he said. 'I think it's just about his favourite spot – you can see how he's enjoying himself.'

I nodded. 'He certainly looks a happy little dog.'

'Yes, he's happy all right. He had a good life and honestly I often forget that he can't see.' He paused. 'You were right, that day in your surgery. You said this would happen.'

'Well, that's great, Andrew,' I said. 'And you're happy, too, aren't you?'

'I am, Mr Herriot. Thank God, I am.' A shadow crossed his face. 'When I think how it was then, I can't believe my luck. It was like being in a dark valley, and bit by bit I've climbed out into the sunshine.'

'I can see that. You're as good as new, now.'

He smiled. 'I'm better than that – better than I was before. That terrible experience did me good. Remember you said I was torturing myself? I realized I had spent all my days doing that. I used to take every little mishap of life and beat myself over the head with it.'

'You don't have to tell me, Andrew,' I said ruefully. 'I've always been pretty good at that myself.'

'Well, yes, I suppose a lot of us are. But I became an expert and see where it got me. It helped so much to have Digger to look after.' His face lit up and he pointed over the grass. 'Just look at that!'

The little dog had been inspecting an ancient fence, a few roting planks which were probably part of an old sheep-fold, and as we watched he leaped effortlessly between the spars to the other side.

'Marvellous!' I said delightedly. 'You'd think there was nothing wrong with him.'

Andrew turned to me. 'Mr Herriot, when I see a thing like that it makes me wonder. Can a blind dog do such a thing. Do you think . . . do you think there's a chance he can see just a little?'

I hesitated. 'Maybe he can see a bit through that pigment, but it can't be much – a flicker of light and shade, perhaps. I really don't know. But in any case, he's become so clever in his familiar surroundings that it doesn't make much difference.'

'Yes . . . yes.' He smiled philosophically. 'Anyway, we must get on our way. Come on, Digger!'

He snapped his fingers and set off along a track which pushed a vivid green finger through the heather, pointing clean and unbroken to the sunny skyline. His dog bounded ahead of him, not just at a trot but at a gallop.

I have made no secret of the fact that I never really knew the cause of Digger's blindness, but in the light of modern developments in eye surgery I believe it was a condition called keratitis sicca. This was simply not recognized in those early days and anyway, if I had known, I could have done little about it. The name means 'dryness of the cornea' and it occurs when the dog is not producing enough tears. At the present time it is treated by instilling artificial tears or by an intricate operation whereby the salivary ducts are transferred to the eyes. But even now, despite these things, I have seen that dread pigmentation taking over in the end.

When I look back on the whole episode my feeling is of thankfulness. All sorts of things help people to pull out of a depression. Mostly it is their family – the knowledge that wife and children are dependent on them – sometimes it is a cause to work for, but in Andrew Vine's case it was a dog.

I often think of the dark valley which closed around him at that time and I am convinced he came out of it on the end of Digger's lead.

14

Now that I had done my first solo I was beginning to appreciate the qualities of my instructor. There was no doubt FO Woodham was a very good teacher.

There was a war on and no time for niceties. He had to get green young men into the air on their own without delay and he had done it with me.

I used to fancy myself as a teacher, too, with the boys who came to see practice in Darrowby. I could see myself now, smiling indulgently at one of my pupils.

'You don't see this sort of thing in country practice, David,' I said. He was one of the young people who occasionally came with me on my rounds. Fifteen years old, and like all the others he thought he wanted to be a veterinary surgeon. But at the moment he looked a little bewildered.

I really couldn't blame him. It was his first visit and he had expected to spend a day with me in the rough and tumble of large animal practice in the Yorkshire Dales and now there was this lady with the poodle and Emmeline. The lady's progress along the passage to the consulting room had been punctuated by a series of squeaking noises produced by her squeezing a small rubber doll. At each squeak Lucy advanced a few reluctant steps until a final pressure lured her on to the table. There she stood trembling and looking soulfully around her.

'She won't go anywhere without Emmeline,' the lady explained.

'Emmeline?'

'The doll.' She held up the rubber toy. 'Since this trouble started Lucy has become devoted to her.'

'I see. And what trouble is that?'

'Well, it's been going on for about two weeks now. She's so listless and strange, and she hardly eats anything.'

I reached behind me to the trolley for the thermometer. 'Right, we'll have a look at her. There's something wrong when a dog won't eat.'

The temperature was normal. I went over her chest thoroughly with my stethoscope without finding any unusual sounds. The heart thudded steadily in my ears. Careful palpation of the abdomen revealed nothing out of the way.

The lady stroked Lucy's curly poll and the little animal looked up at her with sorrowful liquid eyes. 'I'm getting really worried about her. She doesn't want to go walks. In fact we can't even entice her from the house without Emmeline.'

'Eh ?'

'I say she won't take a step outside unless we squeak Emmeline at her, and then they both go out together. Even then she just trails along like an old dog, and she's only three after all. You know how lively she is normally.'

I nodded. I did know. This little poodle was a bundle of energy. I had seen her racing around the fields down by the river, jumping to enormous heights as she chased a ball. She must be suffering from something pretty severe, but so far I was baffled.

And I wished the lady woudn't keep on about Emmeline and the squeaking. I shot a side glance at David. I had been holding forth to him, telling him how ours was a scientific profession and that he would have to be really hot at physics, chemistry and biology to gain entrance to a veterinary school, and it didn't fit in with all this.

Maybe I could guide the conversation along more clinical lines. 'Any more symptoms ?' I asked. 'Any cough, constipation, diarrhoea ? Does she ever cry out in pain ?'

The lady shook her head. 'No, nothing like that. She just moons around looking at us with such a pitiful expression and searching for Emmeline.'

Oh dear, there it was again. I cleared my throat. 'She never vomits at all ? Especially after a meal ?'

'Never. When she does eat a little she goes straight away to find Emmeline and takes her to her basket.'

'Really ? Well I can't see that that has anything to do with it. Are you sure she isn't lame at times ?'

The lady didn't seem to be listening. 'And when she gets Emmeline into her basket she sort of circles around, scratching the blanket as though she was making a bed for the little thing.'

I gritted my teeth. Would she never stop ? Then a light flashed in the darkness.

'Wait a minute,' I said. 'Did you say making a bed?'

'Yes, she scratches around for ages then puts Emmeline down.'

'Ah yes.' The next question would settle it. 'When was she last in season?'

The lady tapped a finger against her cheek. 'Let me see. It was in the middle of May – that would be about nine weeks ago.'

There wasn't a mystery any more.

'Roll her over, please,' I said.

With Lucy stretched on her back, her eyes regarding the surgery ceiling with deep emotion, I ran my fingers over the mammary glands. They were turgid and swollen. I gently squeezed one of the teats and a bead of milk appeared.

'She's got false pregnancy,' I said.

'What on earth is that?' The lady looked at me, round-eyed.

'Oh, it's quite common in bitches. They get the idea they are going to have pups and around the end of the gestation period they start this business. Making a bed for the pups is typical, but some of them actually swell in the abdomen. They do all sorts of peculiar things.'

'My goodness, how extraordinary!' The lady began to laugh. 'Lucy, you silly little thing, worrying us over nothing.' She looked at me across the table. 'How long is she going to be like this?'

I turned on the hot tap and began to wash my hands. 'Not for long. I'll give you some tablets for her. If she's not much better in a week come back for more. But you needn't worry – even if it takes a little bit longer she'll be her old self in the end.'

I went through to the dispensary, put the tablets in a box and handed them over. The lady thanked me then turned to her pet who was sitting on the tiled floor looking dreamily into space.

'Come along, Lucy,' she said, but the poodle took no notice. 'Lucy! Do you hear me? We're going now!' She began to walk briskly along the passage but the little animal merely put her head on one side and appeared to be hearkening to inward music. After a minute her mistress reappeared and regarded her with some exasperation. 'Oh really, you are naughty. I suppose there's only one way.' She opened her handbag and produced the rubber toy.

'Squeak-squeak,' went Emmeline and the poodle raised her eyes with misty adoration. 'Squeak-squeak, squeak-squeak.' The sound retreated along the passage and Lucy followed entranced until she disappeared round the corner.

I turned to David with an apologetic grin. 'Right,' I said, 'we'll get out on the road. I know you want to see farm practice and I assure you it's vastly different from what you've seen here.'

Sitting in the car, I continued. 'Mind you, don't get me wrong. I'm not decrying small animal work. In fact I'd have to admit that it is the most highly skilled branch of the profession and I personally think that small animal surgery is tremendously demanding. Just don't judge it all by Emmeline. Anyway, we have one doggy visit before we go out into the country.'

'What's that ?' the lad asked.

'Well, I've had a call from a Mr Rington to say that his dalmatian bitch has completely altered her behaviour. In fact she's acting so strangely that he doesn't want to bring her to the surgery.'

'What do you think that might be ?'

I thought for a moment. 'It seems a bit silly, but the first thing that comes to my mind is rabies. This is the most dreadful dog disease of all, but thank heaven we've managed to, keep it out of this country so far by strict quarantine regulations. But at college it was hammered into us so forcibly that it is always at the back of my mind even though I don't really expect to see it. But this case of the dalmatian could be anything. I only hope she hasn't turned savage because that's the sort of thing that leads to a dog being put down and I hate that.'

Mr Rington's opening remark didn't cheer me.

'Tessa's become really fierce lately, Mr Herriot. Started moping about and growling a few days ago and frankly I daren't trust her with strangers now. She nailed the postman by the ankle this morning. Most embarrassing.'

My spirits sank lower. 'Actually bit somebody! It's unbelievable – she's such a softie. I've always been able to do anything with her.'

'I know, I know,' he muttered. 'She's marvellous with children, too. I can't understand it. But come and have a look at her.'

The dalmatian was sitting in a corner of the lounge and she glanced up sulkily as we entered. She was a favourite patient and I approached her confidently.

132

'Hello, Tessa,' I said, and held out my hand. I usually had a tail-lashing, tongue-lolling welcome from this animal but today she froze into complete immobility and her lips withdrew silently from her teeth. It wasn't an ordinary snarl – it was as though the upper lip was operated by strings and there was something unnerving about it.

'What's the matter, old girl?' I inquired, and again the gleaming incisors were soundlessly exposed. And as I stared uncomprehendingly I could see that the eyes were glaring at me with blazing primitive hatred. Tessa was unrecognizable.

'Mr Herriot—' Her owner looked at me apprehensively. 'I don't think I'd go any nearer if I were you.'

I withdrew a pace. 'Yes, I'm inclined to agree with you. I don't think she'd cooperate if I tried to examine her. But never mind, tell me all about her.'

'Well, there's really nothing more to tell,' Mr Rington said helpless. 'She's just different – like this.'

'Appetite good?'

'Yes, fine. Eats everything in front of her.'

'No unusual symptoms at all?'

'None, apart from the altered temperament. The family can handle her, but quite frankly I think she'd bite any stranger who came too near.'

I ran my fingers through my hair. 'Any change in family circumstances? New baby? Different domestic help? Unusual people coming to the house?'

'No, nothing like that. There's been no change.'

'I ask because animals sometimes act like this out of jealousy or disapproval.'

'Sorry.' Mr Rington shrugged his shoulders. 'Everything is just as it's always been. Only this morning my wife was wondering if Tessa was still cross with us because we kept her indoors for three weeks while she was in season. But that was a long time ago – about two months now.'

I whipped round and faced him. 'Two months?'

'Yes, about that.'

'Surely not again!' I gestured to the owner. 'Would you please lift her up so that she's standing on her hind legs?'

'Like this?' He put his arms round the dalmatian's chest and

133

hoisted till she was in the upright position with her abdomen facing me.

And it was as if I knew beforehand. Because I felt not the slightest surprise when I saw the twin row of engorged teats. It was unnecessary, but I leaned forward, grasped a little nipple and sent a white jet spurting.

'She's bulging with milk,' I said.

'Milk?'

'Yes, she's got false pregnancy. This is one of the more un-usual side effects, but I'll give you some tablets and she'll soon be the docile Tessa again.'

As we got back into the car I had a good idea what the school-boy was thinking. He would be wondering where the chemistry, physics and biology came in.

'Sorry about that, David,' I said. 'I've been telling you all about the constant variety of a vet's life and the first two cases you see are the same condition. But we are going out to the farms now and, as I said, you'll find it very different. I mean, those two cases were really psychological things. You don't get that in country practice. It's a bit rough but it's real and down to earth.'

As we drove into the farmyard I saw the farmer carrying a bag of meal over the cobbles.

I got out of the car with David. 'You've got a pig ill, Mr Fisher?'

'Aye, a big sow. She's in 'ere.' He led the way into a pen and pointed to a huge white pig lying on her side.

'She's been off it for a few days,' he said. 'Hardly eats owt – just picks at her food. And she just lays there all t'time. Ah don't think she's got strength to get to her feet.'

My thermometer had been in the pig's rectum as he spoke and I fished it out and read the temperature. It was 102.2 – dead normal. I auscultated the chest and palpated the abdomen with growing puzzlement. Nothing wrong. I looked over at the trough nearby. It was filled to the brim with fresh meal and water – untouched. And pigs do love their food.

I nudged her thigh with my fist. 'Come on, lass, get up.' And I followed it with a brisk slap across the rump. A healthy pig would have leaped to her feet but the sow never moved.

I tried not to scratch my head. There was something very funny here. 'Has she ever been ill before, Mr Fisher?'

'Nay, never ailed a thing and she's allus been a real lively pig, too. Ah can't reckon it up.'

Nor could I. 'What beats me,' I said, 'is that she doesn't look like a sick animal. She's not trembling or anxious, she's lying there as if she hadn't a care in the world.'

'Aye, you're right, Mr Herriot. She's as 'appy as Larry, but she'll neither move nor eat. It's a rum 'un, isn't it?'

It was very rum indeed. I squatted on my heels, watching the big sow. She reached forward and pushed gently with her snout at the straw bedding round her head. Sick pigs never did that. It was a gesture of well-being. And those little grunts which issued from deep in her chest. They were grunts of deep contentment and there was something familiar about the sound of them . . . something lurking at the back of my mind which wouldn't come forward. It was the same with the way the sow eased herself further on to her side, pushing the great stretch of abdomen outward as though in offering.

I had heard and seen it so many times before – the happy sounds, the careful movements. Then I remembered. Of course! She was like a sow with a litter, only there was no litter.

A wave of disbelief flowed over me. Oh no, no, please not a third time! It was dark in the pen and I couldn't get a clear view of the mammary glands.

I turned to the farmer. 'Open the door a little will you, please.'

As the sunshine flooded in everything was obvious. It was mere routine to reach out to the long tumefied udder and squirt the milk against the wall.

I straightened up wearily and was about to make my now commonplace announcement when David did it for me.

'False pregnancy?' he said.

I nodded dumbly.

'What was that?' enquired Mr Fisher.

'Well, your sow has got it into her head that she is pregnant,' I said. 'Not only that, but she thinks she has given birth to a litter and she's suckling the imaginary piglets now. You can see it, can't you?'

135

The farmer gave a long soft whistle. 'Aye ... aye ... you're right. That's what she's doin' ... enjoyin' it, too.' He took off his cap, rubbed the top of his head and put the cap on again. 'Well, there's allus summat new, isn't there ?'

It wasn't new to David, of course. Old stuff, in fact, and I didn't want to bore him further with a lengthy dissertation.

'Nothing to worry about, Mr Fisher,' I said hastily. 'Call down to the surgery and I'll give you something to put in her food. She'll soon be back to normal.'

As I left the pen the sow gave a deep sigh of utter fulfilment and moved her position with the utmost care to avoid crushing her phantom family. I looked back at her and I could almost see the long pink row of piglets sucking busily. I shook my head to dispel the vision and went out to the car.

I was opening the door when the farmer's wife trotted towards me. 'I've just had a phone call from your surgery, Mr Herriot. They want you to go to Mr Rogers of East Farm. There's a cow calving.'

An emergency like this in the middle of a round was usually an irritant, but today the news came as a relief. I had promised this schoolboy some genuine country practice and I was beginning to feel embarrassed.

'Well, David,' I said with a light laugh as we drove away. 'You must be thinking all my patients are neurotic. But you're going to see a bit of the real thing now – there's nothing airy-fairy about a calving cow. This is where the hard work of our job comes in. It's often pretty tough fighting against a big straining cow, but you must remember the vet only sees the difficult cases where the calf is laid wrong.'

The situation of East Farm seemed to add weight to my words. We were bumping up the fellside along a narrow track which was never meant for motor cars and I winced as the exhaust grated against the jutting rocks.

The farm was perched almost on the edge of the hilltop and behind it the sparse fields, stolen from the moorland, rolled away to the skyline. The crumbling stonework and broken roof tiles testified to the age of the squat grey house.

I pointed to some figures, faintly visible on the massive stone lintel above the front door. 'What does that date mean to you, David?'

'Sixteen sixty-six, the Great Fire of London,' he replied promptly.

'Well done. Strange to think they were building this place in the same year as old London burned down.'

Mr Rogers appeared, carrying a steaming bucket and a towel. 'She's out in t'field, Mr Herriot, but she's a quiet cow and easy to catch.'

'All right.' I followed him through the gate. It was another little annoyance when the farmer didn't have the cow inside for me but again I felt that if David wanted to be a vet he ought to know that a lot of our work was carried out in the open, often in the cold and rain.

Even now on this July morning a cool breeze whipped round my chest and back as I pulled off my shirt. It was never very warm in the high country of the Dales but I felt at home here. With the cow standing patiently as the farmer held her halter, the bucket perched among the tufts of wiry grass, and only a few stunted wind-bent trees breaking the harsh sweep of green, it seemed that at last this boy was seeing me in my proper place.

I soaped my arms to the shoulders. 'Hold the tail, will you, David. This is where I find out what kind of job it's going to be.'

As I slipped my hand into the cow it struck me that it would be no bad thing if it was a hard calving. If the lad saw me losing a bit of sweat it would give him a truer picture of the life in front of him.

'Sometimes these jobs take an hour or more,' I said. 'But you have the reward of delivering a new living creature. Seeing a calf wriggling on the ground at the end of it is the biggest thrill in practice.'

I reached forward, my mind alive with the possibilities. Posterior? Head back? Breech? But as I groped through the open cervix into the uterus I felt a growing astonishment. There was nothing there.

I withdrew my arm and leaned for a moment on the hairy rump. The day's events were taking on a dreamlike quality. Then I looked up at the farmer.

'There's no calf in this cow, Mr Rogers.'

'Eh?'

'She's empty. She's calved already.'

The farmer gazed around him, scanning the acres of bare grass. 'Well where the hangment is the thing? This cow was messin' about last night and I thought she'd calve, but there was nowt to find this morning'.'

His attention was caught by a cry from the right.

'Hey, Willie! Just a minute, Willie!' It was Bob Sellars from the next farm. He was leaning over the drystone wall about twenty yards away.

'What's matter, Bob?'

'Ah thowt ah'd better tell ye. Ah saw that cow hidin' her calf this morning'.'

'Hidin' ...? What are ye on about?'

'Ah'm not jokin' nor jestin', Willie. She hid it on yon gutter ower there and every time t'calf tried to get out she pushed it back in again.'

'But ... nay, nay, I can't 'ave that. I've never heard of such a thing. Have you, Mr Herriot?'

I shook my head, but the whole thing seemed to fit in with the air of fantasy which had begun to pervade the day's work.

Bob Sellars began to climb over the wall. 'Awright, if ye won't believe me I'll show ye.'

He led the way to the far end of the field where a dry ditch ran along the base of the wall. 'There 'e is!' he said triumphantly.

And there indeed he was. A tiny red and white calf half concealed by the long herbage. He was curled comfortably in his grassy bed, his nose resting on his forelegs.

When the little creature saw his mother he staggered to his feet and clambered shakily up the side of the ditch, but no sooner had he gained the level of the field than the big cow, released now from her halter, lowered her head and gently nudged him back in again.

Bob waved his arm. 'There y'are, she's hidin' it, isn't she?'

Mr Rogers said nothing and I merely shrugged my shoulders, but twice more the calf managed to scramble from the ditch and twice more his mother returned him firmly with her head.

'Well it teks a bit o' believin,' the farmer murmured, half to himself. 'She's had five calves afore this and we've taken 'em straight away from 'er as we allus do. Maybe she wants to keep this 'un for 'erself? I dunno . . . I dunno . . .' His voice trailed away.

Later, as we rattled down the stony track, David turned to me. 'Do you think that cow really hid her calf . . . so that she could keep it for herself?'

I stared helplessly through the glass of the windscreen. 'Well, anybody would tell you it's impossible, but you saw what happened. I'm like Mr Rogers, I just don't know.' I paused as the car dipped into a deep rut and sent us bobbing about. 'But you see some funny things at our job.'

The schoolboy nodded thoughtfully. 'Yes, it seems to me that yours is a funny life altogether.'

15

'Would you care to come and dice with death?'

Flight Lieutenant Cramond looked down at me, his puckish features creased into a mischievous smile. I was sitting at a table in my flying suit waiting to be called for a grading test and I stood up hurriedly.

'You mean . . . go up with you, sir?'

'Yes, that's right.'

'Well, I'm just waiting for . . .'

'Oh I know all about that.' He waved a careless hand. 'But there's no hurry. You've time for a bit of fun first.'

'Just as you say, sir,' I said, and followed him out of the hut. Nobody was quite sure of Flt Lt Cramond's status at the flying school. He wasn't one of the regular instructors – he was a much older man – but he was obviously regarded with respect by his fellow officers and seemed to adopt a freelance role.

He occasionally descended on an unsuspecting trainee pilot with his familiar request, 'Would you care to dice with death?'

and this was invariably followed by a joy ride round the sky, a dazzling display of aerobatics which looked wonderful from the ground but could be shattering in the air.

I had seen pupils tottering green-faced from the Tiger Moth after these sessions, and there seemed to be no particular reason why he did it at all. But there was no doubt he was a brilliant flyer. It was rumoured that he had been a stunt pilot with Alan Cobham's famous air circus, but there were so many rumours in the RAF – like the one about the bromide in the tea – that I never really knew if it was true.

However, I got into the aircraft with a feeling of pleasant anticipation. Whatever happened I wouldn't feel ill, being blessed with a stomach which never got queasy with motion. Over-indulgence can have disastrous effects on my digestive apparatus but otherwise I am immune. I have been on little cattle boats in force nine gales when even the crew were groaning in their bunks, but land-lubber Herriot was still enjoying his four meals a day. It was the same in the air.

I soon had reason to be grateful for this blessing because Flt Lt Cramond threw the little aircraft around the sky in an alarming manner, climbing high, then fluttering earthwards like a falling autumn leaf, doing repeated loops and spins. Most of it I enjoyed because he was a likeable man and the eyes in the mirror were humorous and friendly.

He kept up a running commentary as he went through his repertoire.

'This is Cramond's famous hangover cure,' he announced before going into a violent manoeuvre which involved a lot of flying upside down. To a novice like myself it was a strange sensation to be hanging in my straps, looking up at farmhouses and down at the cloud-strewn sky.

That was the only time I didn't feel too happy, because those canvas straps were attached to the sides of the cockpit by frayed wires which twanged and groaned disturbingly as I hung there. It was a long way to the ground and I kept a hand on the parachute release just in case.

I was wondering how long we were going to stay in this position when he rolled over and went into a long dive. Down and down we roared, heading nose first for the peaceful farm land,

and just as I had concluded that we must certainly plunge straight into the earth he levelled off and we skimmed through a long cornfield with the wheels of the undercarriage trailing among the golden ears.

'This is nice, isn't it ?' Flt Lt Cramond murmured.

And it was nice, too. There was no crop spraying in those days and the scent of the wild flowers growing among the corn drifted into the open cockpit. The heady fragrance took me back in a moment to that picnic with Helen.

There were many things leading up to the picnic. It all started when I caught Helen in the pantry, stealing the porridge oats. She was standing with the packet in her hand, scooping the contents into her mouth with a spoon, and she started guiltily when she saw me.

'You're at it again!' I exclaimed. I snatched the packet from her fingers. 'It's nearly empty! How many do you go through a week ?'

She looked at me with a striken face and shook her head. 'I don't know.'

'But Helen – raw porridge oats! You're not supposed to eat them that way. Not a packet at a time, anyway. You'll give yourself indigestion.'

'I'm all right so far.' Her spoon twitched and I could see she wanted more.

'But why don't you cook them and eat ordinary porridge – do you good that way.'

She pouted. 'Don't want ordinary porridge.'

I gave her an exasperated stare and left her to it. I'd had no experience with pregnant women but I had heard of these cravings and no doubt they were to be respected. With Helen it had started with oranges – oranges morning noon and night – and I was rather pleased because I thought they would be good for her with all those vitamins. But it wasn't long before she went off the oranges and on to the porridge and I started to worry.

However it was needless. Within a week or two the porridge had lost all its attractions and Helen was on the custard. And it was cooked custard, good wholesome stuff made with plenty of milk, and though Helen drank it by the gallon instead of the pint I felt sure it must be beneficial.

The custard phase lasted for some time. Whatever I was doing around our bed-sitter Helen would be crouched over her bowl of custard, imbibing it effortlessly, spoonful by spoonful, watching me with inward-looking eyes. When I was working in the garden I had only to glance up to the little window under the tiles to see that rapt face looking out at me and the spoon rising and falling from the custard bowl.

Such nourishing material, I thought, could do nothing but good both for my wife and for our first born, but before I knew where I was the trouble with the smells began.

It was totally unexpected. We both accepted the fact that our dining arrangements were somewhat primitive. Bare boards, a wooden bench against the wall and a gas ring was all we had. But it was all we wanted, so that it was something of a shock to me when Helen complained.

It was one lunchtime and she looked around her, sniffing suspiciously. 'There's a funny smell in here,' she said.

'A funny smell? What do you mean?' I was utterly at a loss because just about the only thing that annoyed me about my new wife was that she spent far too much time scrubbing and cleaning our premises. There just couldn't be any smells.

But it began to happen every day. Each lunchtime when we climbed the long flights of stairs to our kitchen Helen's nose began to wrinkle almost as soon as the door closed behind her. Matters came to a head at the end of a week.

'Jim,' she said mournfully. 'I can't eat here any more. Not with this smell about.'

It was a problem. Lunch was our main meal of the day and she had almost stopped eating breakfast. Also, the reassuring consumption of custard had dwindled. If this went on she would suffer from malnutrition. Then I had one of my infrequent ideas.

'Let's go out to lunch,' I said.

'Where?'

'The Lilac Café. They say it's very good.'

She nodded uncertainly. 'All right, we'll try it. I just can't eat up here, anyway.'

For a couple of weeks I was sure the problem was solved. The food at the Lilac was excellent and didn't put any strain on our limited financial resources. You could get soup, meat, potatoes and two veg, apple pie and cream, coffee and biscuits all for one and sixpence. Helen enjoyed it all and I was triumphant.

It was only on market days that the Lilac was full, with the farmers and their wives packing the place, and it was on a market day that the blow fell. I was sipping my coffee and making conversation with two stout ladies at the next table when my wife nudged me.

'Jim,' she whispered, and I felt a premonition as I saw the familiar hunted look on her face. 'There's a funny smell in here.'

I stared at her. 'What kind of smell – the same as the one at home?'

'No.' She shook her head miserably. 'But it's funny.'

'But Helen, this is pure imagination.' I raised my head and gave a few ostentatious sniffs. 'There's nothing here at all.'

But she was already on her way out and I realized with a sense of loss that that was the end of the Lilac.

For the next few days we tried the Dickon Street Café. It was much smaller and the food was definitely uninspiring but Helen seemed content, so I was thankful. After all, I told myself as I chewed at a toughish piece of rump steak, she was the one who was having the baby and it was only right that I should humour her. And I was just thinking that matters could be a lot worse when she leaned across the table.

'Can't you smell it?' she asked, wide-eyed.

I felt a surge of despair. 'Smell what?'

'That funny smell. Surely you must be able to . . .' She gazed at me appealingly.

'No, I can't,' I said. 'But never mind, we'll try somewhere else tomorrow.'

Darrowby didn't run to many cafés and there was only one left. It was known simply as Mrs Ackerley's and consisted of one tiny room in that lady's house down a side street. The cuisine there was frankly sub-standard and Mrs Ackerley herself didn't seem to have much faith in its because she invariably added 'Praps not' to every suggestion.

'Would you like some liver – or praps not? Or some toad-in-the-hole – or praps not?' Then for dessert it would be the same. 'How about prunes and rice – or praps not?'

Everything was badly cooked and yet it fascinated me that she

143

had her faithful clientele; an old man who worked at the shoe shop, a middle-aged spinster school teacher and a pale dyspeptic-looking young man whom I recognized as a clerk from the bank. They came every day and I realized I was exploring a hitherto unknown stratum of Darrowby society.

Helen seemed to find some humour in the situation. 'Let's get round to Praps Not's,' she would say each day and I hoped this was a good sign. But I could not stifle the lurking conviction within me that Mrs Ackerley wouldn't last.

I was pushing some particularly tired-looking cabbage round my plate when I heard a sharp intake of breath. My wife was sitting bolt upright, snuffing the air like a hound on the scent.

'Jim,' she muttered urgently, 'There's a . . .'

I held up a hand. 'Okay, okay, you don't have to tell me. Let's go.'

Our position was critical. We had run out of cafés and yet we couldn't live without eating. It was Helen who found the answer.

'It's lovely weather,' she said, slipping her arm through mine. 'Let's have a picnic tomorrow.'

One thing about living in Darrowby is that you don't have to drive very far to leave the town behind. Next day we sat down on a grassy bank and as we opened our packet of sandwiches the September sun flooded down, warming the grey stones of the wall behind us, slanting dazzlingly against the tumbling water of the river far below.

Beyond the wall lay the wide golden sweep of a cornfield and a little breeze stirred the ripe ears into a long slow whisper, bringing with it the sweet scent of a thousand growing things.

Helen sliced a tomato, shook some salt on to it and drew a long contented breath.

'Nice smell here,' she said.

16

The doctor put down the folder containing my case history and gave me a friendly smile across the desk.

'I'm sorry, Herriot, but you've got to have an operation.'

His words, though gentle, were like a slap in the face. After flying school we had been posted to Heaton Park, Manchester, and I heard within two days that I had been graded pilot. Everything seemed at last to be going smoothly.

'An operation . . . are you sure?'

'Absolutely, I'm afraid,' he said, and he looked like a man who knew his business. He was a Wing Commander, almost certainly a specialist in civilian life, and I had been sent to him after a medical inspection by one of the regular doctors.

'This old surgical scar they mention in your documents,' he went on. 'You've already had surgery there, haven't you?'

'Yes, a few years ago.'

'Well, I'm afraid the thing is opening up again and needs attention.'

I seemed to have run out of words and could think of only one.
'When?'

'Immediately. Within a few days, anyway.'

I stared at him. 'But my flight's going overseas at the end of the week.'

'Ah well, that's a pity.' He spread his hands and smiled again. 'But they'll be going without you. You will be in hospital.'

I had a sudden feeling of loss, of something coming to an end, and it lingered after I had left the Wing Commander's office. I realized painfully that the fifty men with whom I had sweated my way through all those new experiences had become my friends. The first breaking-in at St John's Wood in London, the hard training at Scarborough ITW, the 'toughening course' in Shropshire and the final flying instruction at Winkfield; it had bound us together and I had come to think of myself not as an individual but as part of a group. My mind could hardly accept the fact that I was going to be on my own.

The others were sorry, too, my own particular chums looking

almost bereaved, but they were all too busy to pay me much attention. They were being pushed around all over the place, getting briefed and kitted out for their posting, and it was a hectic time for the whole flight – except me. I sat on my bed in the Nissen hut while the excitement billowed around me.

I thought my departure would go unnoticed but when I got my summons and prepared to leave I found, tucked in the webbing of my pack, an envelope filled with the precious coupons with which we drew our ration of cigarettes in those days. It seemed that nearly everybody had chipped in and the final gesture squeezed at my throat as I made my lonely way from the camp.

The hospital was at Creden Hill, near Hereford, and I suppose it is one of the consolations of service life that you can't feel lonely for very long. The beds in the long ward were filled with people like myself who had been torn from their comrades and were eager to be friendly.

In the few days before my operation we came to know each other pretty well. The young man in the bed on my left spent his time writing excruciating poetry to his girlfriend and insisted on reading it out to me, stanza by stanza. The lad on the right seemed a pensive type. Everybody addressed him as 'Sammy' but he replied only in grunts.

When he found out I was a vet he leaned from the sheets and beckoned to me.

'I got fed up wi' them blokes callin' me Sammy,' he muttered in a ripe Birmingham accent. 'Because me name's not Sammy, it's Desmond.'

'Really? Why do they do it, then?'

He leaned out further. 'That's what I want to talk to you about. You bein' a vet – you'll know about these things. It's because of what's wrong with me – why I'm in 'ere.'

'Well, why are you here? What's your trouble?'

He looked around him then spoke in a confidential whisper. 'I gotta big ball.'

'A what?'

'A big ball. One of me balls is a right whopper.'

'Ah, I see, but I still don't understand . . .'

'Well, it's like this,' he said. 'All the fellers in the ward keep

146

sayin' the doctor's goin' to cut it off – then I'd be like Sammy Hall.'

I nodded in comprehension. Memories from my college days filtered back. It had been a popular ditty at the parties. 'My name is Sammy Hall and I've only got one ball . . .'

'Oh, nonsense, they're pulling your leg,' I said. 'An enlarged testicle can be all sorts of things. Can you remember what the doctor called it ?'

He screwed up his face. 'It was a funny name. Like vorry or varry something.'

'Do you mean varicocele ?'

'That's it!' He threw up an arm. 'That's the word!'

'Well, you can stop worrying,' I said. 'It's quite a simple little operation. Trifling, in fact.'

'You mean they won't cut me ball off ?'

'Definitely not. Just remove a few surplus blood vessels, that's all. No trouble.'

He fell back on the pillow and gazed ecstatically at the ceiling. 'Thanks, mate,' he breathed. 'You've done me a world o' good. I'm gettin' done tomorrow and I've been dreadin' it.'

He was like a different person all that day, laughing and joking with everybody, and next morning when the nurse came to give him his pre-med injection he turned to me with a last appeal in his eyes.

'You wouldn't kid me, mate, would you ? They're not goin' to . . . ?'

I held up a hand. 'I assure you, Sammy – er – Desmond, you've nothing to worry about. I give you my word.'

Again the beatific smile crept over his face and it stayed there until the 'blood wagon', the operating room trolley, pushed by a male orderly, came to collect him.

The blood wagon was very busy each morning and it was customary to raise a cheer as each man was wheeled out. Most of the victims responded with a sleepy wave before the swing doors closed behind them, but when I saw Desmond grinning cheerfully and giving the thumbs-up sign I felt I had really done something.

Next morning it was my turn. I had my injection at around eight o'clock and by the time the trolley appeared I was pleasantly woozy. They removed my pyjamas and arrayed me in a sort of nightgown with laces at the neck and pulled thick woollen socks over my feet. As the orderly wheeled me away the inmates of the ward broke into a ragged chorus of encouragement and I managed the ritual flourish of an arm as I left.

It was a cheerless journey along white-tiled corridors until the trolley pushed its way into the anaesthetics room. As I entered, the doors at the far end parted as a doctor came towards me bearing a loaded syringe. I had a chilling glimpse of the operating theatre beyond, with the lights beating on the long table and the masked surgeons waiting.

The doctor pushed up my sleeve and swabbed my forearm with surgical spirit. I decided I had seen enough and closed my eyes, but an exclamation from above made me open them.

'Good God, it's Jim Herriot!'

I looked up at the man with the syringe. It was Teddy McQueen. He had been in my class at school and I hadn't seen him since the day I left.

My throat was dry after the injection but I felt I had to say something.

'Hello, Teddy,' I croaked.

His eyes were wide. 'What the hell are you doing here ?'

'What the hell do you think ?' I rasped crossly. 'I'm going in there for an operation.'

'Oh, I know that – I'm the anaesthetist here – but I remember you telling me at school that you were going to be a vet.'

'That's right. I am a vet.'

'You are ?' His face was a picture of amazement. 'But what the devil is a vet doing in the RAF ?'

It was a good question. 'Nothing very much, Teddy,' I replied.

He began to laugh. Obviously he found the whole situation intriguing.

'Well, Jim, I can't get over this!' He leaned over me and giggled uncontrollably. 'Imagine our meeting here after all these years. I think it's an absolute hoot!' His whole body began to shake and he had to dab away the tears from his eyes.

Lying there on the blood wagon in my nightie and woolly socks I didn't find it all that funny, and my numbed brain was searching for a withering riposte when a voice barked from the theatre.

'What's keeping you, McQueen? We can't wait all morning!'

Teddy stopped laughing. 'Sorry, Jim, old chum,' he said. 'But your presence is requested within.' He pushed the needle into my vein and my last memory as I drifted away was of his lingering amused smile.

I spent three weeks at Creden Hill and towards the end of that time those of us who were almost fully recovered were allowed out to visit the nearby town of Hereford. This was embarrassing because we were all clad in the regulation suit of hospital blue with white shirt and red tie and it was obvious from the respectful glances we received that people thought we had been wounded in action.

When a veteran of the First World War came up to me and asked, 'Where did you get your packet, mate?' I stopped going altogether.

I left the RAF hospital with a feeling of gratitude – particularly towards the hard-working, cheerful nurses. They gave us many a tongue lashing for chattering after lights out, for smoking under the blankets, for messing up our beds, but all the time I marvelled at their dedication.

I used to lie there and wonder what it was in a girl's character that made her go in for the arduous life of nursing. A concern for people's welfare? A natural caring instinct? Whatever it was, I was sure a person was born with it.

This trait is part of the personalities of some animals and it was exemplified in Eric Abbot's sheepdog, Judy.

I first met Judy when I was treating Eric's bullock for wooden tongue. The bullock was only a young one and the farmer admitted ruefully that he had neglected it because it was almost a walking skeleton.

'Damn!' Eric grunted. 'He's been runnin' out with that bunch in the far fields and I must have missed 'im. I never knew he'd got to this state.'

When actinobacillosis affects the tongue it should be treated right at the start, when the first symptoms of salivation and swelling beneath the jaw appear. Otherwise the tongue becomes harder and harder till finally it sticks out of the front of the mouth, as unyielding as the wood which gives the disease its ancient name.

This skinny little creature had reached that state, so that he not only looked pathetic but also slightly comic as though he were making a derisive gesture at me. But with a tongue like that he just couldn't eat and was literally starving to death. He lay quietly as though he didn't care.

'There's one thing, Eric,' I said. 'Giving him an intravenous injection won't be any problem. He hasn't the strength to resist.'

The great new treatment at that time was sodium iodide into the vein – modern and spectacular. Before that the farmers used to paint the tongue with tincture of iodine, a tedious procedure which sometimes worked and sometimes didn't. The sodium iodide was a magical improvement and showed results within a few days.

I inserted the needle into the jugular and tipped up the bottle of clear fluid. Two drachms of the iodide I used to use, in eight ounces of distilled water and it didn't take long to flow in. In fact the bottle was nearly empty before I noticed Judy.

I had been aware of a big dog sitting near me all the time, but as I neared the end of the injection a black nose moved ever closer till it was almost touching the needle. Then the nose moved along the rubber tube up to the bottle and back again, sniffing with the utmost concentration. When I removed the needle the nose began a careful inspection of the injection site. Then a tongue appeared and began to lick the bullock's neck methodically.

I squatted back on my heels and watched. This was something more than mere curiosity; everything in the dog's attitude suggested intense interest and concern.

'You know, Eric,' I said. 'I have the impression that this dog isn't just watching me. She's supervising the whole job.'

The farmer laughed. 'You're right there. She's a funny old bitch is Judy – sort of a nurse. If there's anything amiss she's on duty. You can't keep her away.'

Judy looked up quickly at the sound of her name. She was a handsome animal; not the usual colour, but a variegated brindle with waving lines of brown and grey mingling with the normal black and white of the farm collie. Maybe there was a cross somewhere but the result was very attractive and the effect was heightened by her bright-eyed, laughing-mouthed friendliness.

I reached out and tickled the backs of her ears and she wagged mightily – not just her tail but her entire rear end. 'I suppose she's just good-natured.'

'Oh aye, she is,' the farmer said. 'But it's not only that. It sounds daft but I think Judy feels a sense of responsibility to all the stock on t'farm.'

I nodded. 'I believe you. Anyway, let's get this beast on to his chest.'

We got down in the straw and with our hands under the backbone, rolled the bullock till he was resting on his sternum. We balanced him there with straw bales on either side then covered him with a horse rug.

In that position he didn't look as moribund as before, but the emaciated head with the useless jutting tongue lolled feebly on his shoulders and the saliva drooled uncontrolled on to the straw. I wondered if I'd ever see him alive again.

Judy however didn't appear to share my pessimism. After a thorough sniffing examination of rug and bales she moved to the front, applied an encouraging tongue to the shaggy forehead then stationed herself comfortably facing the bullock, very like a night nurse keeping an eye on her patient.

'Will she stay there?' I closed the half-door and took a last look inside.

'Aye, nothing'll shift her till he's dead or better,' Eric replied. 'She's in her element now.'

'Well, you never know, she may give him an interest in life, just sitting there. He certainly needs some help. You must keep him alive with milk or gruel till the injection starts to work. If he'll drink it it'll do him most good but otherwise you'll have to bottle it into him. But be careful – you can choke a beast that way.'

A case like this had more than the usual share of the old fascination because I was using a therapeutic agent which really worked – something that didn't happen too often at that time. So I was eager to get back to see if I had been able to pull that bullock from the brink of death. But I knew I had to give the drug a chance and kept away for five days.

When I walked across the yard to the box I knew there would be no further doubts. He would either be dead or on the road to recovery.

The sound of my steps on the cobbles hadn't gone unnoticed. Judy's head, ears cocked, appeared above the half-door. A little well of triumph brimmed in me. If the nurse was still on duty then the patient must be alive. And I felt even more certain when the big dog disappeared for a second, then came soaring effortlessly over the door and capered up to me, working her hind end into convolutions of delight. She seemed to be doing her best to tell me all was well.

Inside the box the bullock was still lying down but he turned to look at me and I noticed a strand of hay hanging from his mouth. The tongue itself had disappeared behind the lips.

'Well, we're winnin', aren't we?' Eric Abbot came in from the yard.

'Without a doubt,' I said. 'The tongue's much softer and I see he's been trying to eat hay.'

'Aye, can't quite manage it yet, but he's suppin' the milk and gruel like a good 'un. He's been up a time or two but he's very wobbly on his pins.'

I produced another bottle of sodium iodide and repeated the injection with Judy's nose again almost touching the needle as she sniffed avidly. Her eyes were focused on the injection site with fierce concentration and so intent was she on extracting the full savour that she occasionally blew out her nostrils with a sharp blast before recommencing her inspection.

When I had finished she took up her position at the head and as I prepared to leave I noticed a voluptuous swaying of her hips which were embedded in the straw. I was a little puzzled until I realized she was wagging in the sitting position.

'Well, Judy's happy at the way things are going,' I said.

The farmer nodded. 'Yes, she is. She likes to be in charge. Do you know, she gives every newborn calf a good lick over as soon as it comes into t'world and it's the same whenever one of our cats 'as kittens.'

'Bit of a midwife, too, eh ?'

'You could say that. And another funny thing about 'er – she lives with the livestock in the buildings. She's got a nice warm kennel but she never bothers with it – sleeps with the beasts in the straw every night.'

I revisited the bullock a week later and this time he galloped round the box like a racehorse when I approached him. When I finally trapped him in a corner and caught his nose I was breathless but happy. I slipped my fingers into his mouth; the tongue was pliable and almost normal.

'One more shot, Eric', I said. 'Wooden tongue is the very devil for recurring if you don't get it cleared up thoroughly.' I began to unwind the rubber tube. 'By the way, I don't see Judy around.'

'Oh, I reckon she feels he's cured now, and anyway, she has summat else on her plate this mornin'. Can you see her over there ?'

I looked through the doorway. Judy was stalking importantly across the yard. She had something in her mouth – a yellow fluffy object.

I craned out further. 'What is she carrying ?'

'It's a chicken.'

'A chicken ?'

'Aye, there's a brood of them runnin' around just now. They're only a month old and t'awd bitch seems to think they'd be better off in the stable. She's made a bed for them in there and she keeps tryin' to curl herself round them. But the little things won't 'ave it.'

I watched Judy disappear into the stable. Very soon she came out, trotted after a group of tiny chicks which were pecking happily among the cobbles and gently scooped one up. Busily she made her way back to the stable but as she entered the previous chick reappeared in the doorway and pottered over to rejoin his friends.

She was having a frustrating time but I knew she would keep at it because that was the way she was.

Judy, the nurse dog, was still on duty.

17

My experience in the RAF hospital made me think. As a veterinary surgeon I had become used to being on the other end of the knife and I preferred it that way.

As I remembered, I was quite happy that morning a couple of years ago as I poised my knife over a swollen ear. Tristan, one elbow leaning wearily on the table, was holding an anaesthetic mask over the nose of the sleeping dog when Siegfried came into the room.

He glanced briefly at the patient. 'Ah yes, that haematoma you were telling me about, James.' Then he looked across the table at his brother. 'Good God, you're a lovely sight this morning! When did you get in last night?'

Tristan raised a pallid countenance. He eyes were bloodshot slits between puffy lids. 'Oh, I don't quite know. Fairly late, I should think.'

'Fairly late! I got back from a farrowing at four o'clock and you hadn't arrived then. Where the hell were you, anyway?'

'I was at the Licensed Victuallers' Ball. Very good do, actually.'

'I bet it was!' Siegfried snorted. 'You don't miss a thing, do you? Darts Team Dinner, Bellringers' Outing, Pigeon Club Dance and now it's the Licensed Victuallers' Ball. If there's a good booze-up going on anywhere you'll find it.'

When under fire Tristan always retained his dignity and he drew it around him now like a threadbare cloak.

'As a matter of fact,' he said, 'many of the Licensed Victuallers are my friends.'

His brother flushed. 'I believe you. I should think you're the best bloody customer they've ever had!'

Tristan made no reply but began to make a careful check of the flow of oxygen into the ether bottle.

'And another thing,' Siegfried continued. 'I keep seeing you slinking around with about a dozen different women. And you're supposed to be studying for an exam.'

'That's an exaggeration.' The young man gave him a pained

look. 'I admit I enjoy a little female company now and then – just like yourself.'

Tristan believed in attack as the best form of defence, and it was a telling blow because there was a constant stream of attractive girls laying siege to Siegfried at Skeldale House.

But the elder brother was only temporarily halted. 'Never mind me!' he shouted. 'I've passed all my exams. I'm talking about you! Didn't I see you with that new barmaid from the Drovers' the other night? You dodged rapidly into a shop doorway but I'm bloody sure it was you.'

Tristan cleared his throat. 'It quite possibly was. I have recently become friendly with Lydia – she's a very nice girl.'

'I'm not saying she isn't. What I am saying is that I want to see you indoors at night with your books instead of boozing and chasing women. Is that clear?'

'Quite.' The young man inclined his head gracefully and turned down the knob on the anaesthetic machine.

His brother regarded him balefully for a few moments, breathing deeply. These remonstrations always took it out of him. Then he turned away quickly and left.

Tristan's façade crumbled as soon as the door closed.

'Watch the anaesthetic for a minute, Jim,' he croaked. He went over to the basin in the corner, filled a measuring jar with cold water and drank it at a long gulp. Then he soaked some cotton wool under the tap and applied it to his brow.

'I wish he hadn't come in just then. I'm in no mood for the raised voices and angry words.' He reached up to a large bottle of aspirins, swallowed a few and washed them down with another gargantuan draught. 'All right then, Jim,' he murmured as he returned to the table and took over the mask again. 'Let's go.'

I bent once more over the sleeping dog. He was a Scottie called Hamish and his mistress, Miss Westerman, had brought him in two days ago.

She was a retired school teacher and I always used to think she must have had little trouble in keeping her class in order. The chilly pale eyes looking straight into mine reminded me that she was as tall as I was and the square jaw between the muscular shoulders completed a redoubtable presence.

'Mr Herriot,' she barked. 'I want you to have a look at Hamish. I do hope it's nothing serious but his ear has become very swollen and painful. They don't get – er – cancer there, do they?' For a moment the steady gaze wavered.

'Oh, that's most unlikely.' I lifted the little animal's chin and looked at the left ear which was drooping over the side of his face. His whole head, in fact, was askew as though dragged down by pain.

Carefully I lifted the ear and touched the tense swelling with a forefinger. Hamish looked round at me and whimpered.

'Yes, I know, old chap. It's tender, isn't it?' As I turned to Miss Westerman I almost bumped into the close-cropped iron-grey head which was hovering close over the little dog.

'He's got an aural haematoma,' I said.

'What on earth is that?'

'It's when the little blood vessels between the skin and cartilage of the ear rupture and the blood flows out and causes this acute distension.'

She patted the jet black shaggy coat. 'But what causes it?'

'Canker, usually. Has he been shaking his head lately?'

'Yes, now you mention it he has. Just as though he had got something in his ear and was trying to get rid of it.'

'Well that's what bursts the blood vessels. I can see he has a touch of canker though it isn't common in this breed.'

She nodded. 'I see. And how can you cure it?'

'Only by an operation, I'm afraid.'

'Oh dear!' She put her hand to her mouth. 'I'm not keen on that.'

'That's nothing to worry about,' I said. 'It's just a case of letting the blood out and stitching the layers of the ear together. If we don't do this soon he'll suffer a lot of pain and finish up with a cauliflower ear, and we don't want that because he's a bonny little chap.'

I meant it, too. Hamish was a proud-strutting, trim little dog. The Scottish terrier is an attractive creature and I often lament that there are so few around in these modern days.

After some hesitation Miss Westerman agreed and we fixed a date two days from then. When she brought him in for the operation she deposited Hamish in my arms, stroked his head again and again, then looked from Tristan to me and back again.

'You'll take care of him, won't you,' she said, and the jaw jutted and the pale blue eyes stabbed. For a moment I felt like a little boy caught in mischief, and I think my colleague felt the same because he blew out his breath as the lady departed.

'By gum, Jim, that's a tough baby,' he muttered. 'I wouldn't like to get on the wrong side of her.'

I nodded. 'Yes, and she thinks all the world of this dog, so let's make a good job of him.'

After Siegfried's departure I lifted the ear which was now a turgid cone and made an incision along the inner skin. As the pent up blood gushed forth I caught it in an enamel dish, then I squeezed several big clots through the wound.

'No wonder the poor little chap was in pain,' I said softly. 'He'll feel a lot better when he wakes up.'

I filled the cavity between skin and cartilage with sulphanilamide then began to stitch the layers together, using a row of buttons. You had to do something like this or the thing filled up again within a few days. When I first began to operate on aural haematomata I used to pack the interior with gauze, then bandage the ear to the head. The owners often made little granny-hats to try to keep the bandage in place, but a frisky dog usually had it off very soon.

The buttons were a far better idea and kept the layers in close contact, lessening the chance of distortion.

By lunchtime Hamish had come round from the anaesthetic and though still slightly dopey he already seemed to be relieved that his bulging ear had been deflated. Miss Westerman had gone away for the day and was due to pick him up in the evening. The little dog, curled in his basket, waited philosophically.

At teatime, Siegfried glanced across the table at his brother. 'I'm going off to Brawton for a few hours, Tristan,' he said. 'I want you to stay in the house and give Miss Westerman her dog when she arrives. I don't know just when she'll come.' He scooped out a spoonful of jam. 'You can keep an eye on the patient and do a bit of studying, too. It's about time you had a night at home.'

Tristan nodded. 'Right, I'll do that.' But I could see he wasn't enthusiastic.

When Siegfried had driven away Tristan rubbed his chin and gazed reflectively through the french window into the darkening garden. 'This is distinctly awkward, Jim.'

'Why?'

'Well, Lydia has tonight off and I promised to see her.' He whistled a few bars under his breath. 'It seems a pity to waste the opportunity just when things are building up nicely. I've got a strong feeling that girl fancies me. In fact she's nearly eating out of my hand.'

I looked at him wonderingly. 'My God, I thought you'd want a bit of peace and quiet and an early bed after last night!'

'Not me,' he said. 'I'm raring to go again.'

And indeed he looked fresh and fit, eyes sparkling, roses back in his cheeks.

'Look, Jim,' he went on. 'I don't suppose you could stick around with this dog?'

I shrugged. 'Sorry, Triss. I'm going back to see that cow of Ted Binns' – right at the top of the Dale. I'll be away for nearly two hours.'

For a few moments he was silent, then he raised a finger. 'I think I have the solution. It's quite simple, in fact it's perfect. I'll bring Lydia in here.'

'What! Into the house?'

'Yes, into this very room. I can put Hamish in his basket by the fire and Lydia and I can occupy the sofa. Marvellous! What could be nicer on a cold winter's night. Cheap, too.'

'But Triss! How about Siegfried's lecture this morning? What if he comes home early and catches the two of you here?'

Tristan lit a Woodbine and blew out an expansive cloud. 'Not a chance. You worry about such tiny things, Jim. He's always late when he goes to Brawton. There's no problem at all.'

'Well, please yourself,' I said. 'But I think you're asking for trouble. Anyway, shouldn't you be doing a bit of bacteriology? The exams are getting close.'

He smiled seraphically through the smoke. 'Oh, I'll have a quick read through it all in good time.'

I couldn't argue with him there. I always had to go over a thing about six times before it finally sank in, but with his brain the quick read would no doubt suffice. I went out on my call.

I got back about eight o'clock and as I opened the front door my mind was far from Tristan. Ted Binns's cow wasn't responding to my treatment and I was beginning to wonder if I was on the right track. When in doubt I liked to look the subject up and the books were on the shelves in the sitting room. I hurried along the passage and threw open the door.

For a moment I stood there bewildered, trying to reorientate my thoughts. The sofa was drawn close to the bright fire, the atmosphere was heavy with cigarette smoke and the scent of perfume, but there was nobody to be seen.

The most striking feature was the long curtain over the french window. It was wafting slowly downwards as though some object had just hurtled through it at great speed. I trotted over the carpet and peered out into the dark garden. From somewhere in the gloom I heard a scuffling noise, a thud and a muffled cry, then there was a pitter-patter followed by a shrill yelping. I stood for some time listening, then as my eyes grew accustomed to the darkness I walked down the long path under the high brick wall to the yard at the foot. The yard door was open as were the big double doors into the back lane, but there was no sign of life.

Slowly I retraced my steps to the warm oblong of light at the foot of the tall old house. I was about to close the french window when I heard a stealthy movement and an urgent whisper.

'Is that you, Jim?'

'Triss! Where the hell have you sprung from?'

The young man tiptoed past me into the room and looked around him anxiously. 'It was you, then, not Siegfried?'

'Yes, I've just come in.'

He flopped on the sofa and sunk his head in his hands. 'Oh damn! I was just lying here a few minutes ago with Lydia in my arms. At peace with the world. Everything was wonderful. Then I heard the front door open.'

'But you knew I was coming back.'

'Yes, and I'd have given you a shout, but for some reason I thought, "God help us, it's Siegfried!" It sounded like his step in the passage.'

'Then what happened?'

He churned his hair around with his fingers. 'Oh, I panicked. I was whispering lovely things into Lydia's ear, then the next second I grabbed her, threw her off the couch and out of the french window.'

'I heard a thud ...'

'Yes, that was Lydia falling into the rockery.'

'And then some sort of high-pitched cries ...'

He signed and closed his eyes. 'That was Lydia in the rose bushes. She doesn't know the geography of the place, poor lass.'

'Gosh, Triss,' I said. 'I'm really sorry. I shouldn't have burst in on you like that. I was thinking of something else.'

He rose wearily and put a hand on my shoulder. 'Not your fault, Jim, not your fault. You did warn me.' He reached for his cigarettes. 'I don't know how I'm going to face that girl again. I just chucked her out into the lane and told her to beat it home with all speed. She must think I'm stone barmy.' He gave a hollow groan.

I tried to be cheerful. 'Oh, you'll get round her again. You'll have a laugh about it later.'

But he wasn't listening. His eyes, wide with horror, were staring past me. Slowly he raised a trembling finger and pointed towards the fireplace. His mouth worked for a few seconds before he spoke.

'Christ, Jim, it's gone!' he gasped.

For a moment I thought the shock had deranged him. 'Gone ...? What's gone?'

'The bloody dog! He was there when I dashed outside. Right there!'

I looked down at the empty basket and a cold hand clutched at me. 'Oh no! He must have got out through the open window. We're in trouble.'

We rushed into the garden and searched in vain. We came back for torches and searched once more, prowling around the yard and back lane, shouting the little dog's name with diminishing hope.

After ten minutes we trailed back to the brightly lit room and stared at each other.

Tristan was the first to voice our thoughts. 'What do we tell Miss Westerman when she calls?'

I shook my head. My mind fled from the thought of informing that lady that we had lost her dog.

Just at that moment the front door bell pealed in the passage and Tristan almost leaped in the air.

'Oh God!' he quavered. 'That'll be her now. Go and see her, Jim. Tell her it was my fault – anything you like – but I daren't face her.'

I squared my shoulders, marched over the long stretch of tiles and opened the door. It wasn't Miss Westerman, it was a well-built platinum blonde and she glared at me angrily.

'Where's Tristan?' she rasped in a voice which told me we had more than one tough female to deal with tonight.

'Well, he's – er—.'

'Oh, I know he's in there!' As she brushed past me I noticed she had a smear of soil on her cheek and her hair was sadly disarranged. I followed her into the room where she stalked up to my friend.

'Look at my bloody stockings!' she burst out. 'They're ruined!'

Tristan peered nervously at the shapely legs. 'I'm sorry, Lydia. I'll get you another pair. Honestly, love, I will.'

'You'd better, you bugger!' she replied. 'And don't "love" me – I've never been so insulted in my life. What did you think you were playing at?'

'It was all a misunderstanding. Let me explain . . .' Tristan advanced on her with a brave attempt at a winning smile, but she backed away.

'Keep your distance,' she said frigidly. 'I've had enough of you for one night.'

She swept out and Tristan leaned his head against the mantelpiece. 'The end of a lovely friendship, Jim.' Then he shook himself. 'But we've got to find that dog. Come on.'

I set off in one direction and he went in the other. It was a moonless night of impenetrable darkness and we were looking for a jet black dog. I think we both knew it was hopeless but we had to try.

In a little town like Darrowby you are soon out on the country roads where there are no lights and as I stumbled around peering vainly over invisible fields the utter pointlessness of the activity became more and more obvious.

Occasionally I came within Tristan's orbit and heard his despairing cries echoing over the empty landscape. 'Haamiish! Haamiish! Haamiish ... !'

After half an hour we met at Skeldale House. Tristan faced me and as I shook my head he seemed to shrink within himself. His chest heaved as he fought for breath. Obviously he had been running while I had been walking and I suppose that was natural enough. We were both in an awkward situation but the final devastating blow would inevitably fall on him.

'Well, we'd better get out on the road again,' he gasped, and as he spoke the front door bell rang again.

The colour drained rapidly from his face and he clutched my arm. 'That must be Miss Westerman this time. God almighty, she's coming in!'

Rapid footsteps sounded in the passage and the sitting room door opened. But it wasn't Miss Westerman, it was Lydia again. She strode over to the sofa, reached underneath and extracted her handbag. She didn't say anything but merely shrivelled Tristan with a sidelong glance before leaving.

'What a night!' he moaned, putting a hand to his forehead. 'I can't stand much more of this.'

Over the next hour we made innumerable sorties but we couldn't find Hamish and nobody else seemed to have seen him. I came in to find Tristan collapsed in an armchair. His mouth hung open and he showed every sign of advanced exhaustion. I shook my head and he shook his then I heard the telephone.

I lifted the receiver, listened for a minute and turned to the young man. 'I've got to go out, Triss. Mr Drew's old pony has colic again.'

He reached out a hand from the depth of his chair. 'You're not going to leave me, Jim?'

'Sorry, I must. But I won't be long. It's only a mile away.'

'But what if Miss Westerman comes?'

I shrugged. 'You'll just have to apologize. Hamish is bound to turn up – maybe in the morning.'

'You make it sound easy ...' He ran a hand inside his collar. 'And another thing – how about Siegfried? What if he arrives and asks about the dog? What do I tell him?'

'Oh, I shouldn't worry about that.' I replied airily. 'Just say you were too busy on the sofa with the Drovers' barmaid to bother about such things. He'll understand.'

But my attempt at jocularity fell flat. The young man fixed me with a cold eye and ignited a quivering Woodbine. 'I believe I've told you this before, Jim, but there's a nasty cruel streak in you.'

Mr Drew's pony had almost recovered when I got there but I gave it a mild sedative injection before turning for home. On the way back a thought struck me and I took a road round the edge of the town to the row of modern bungalows where Miss Westerman lived. I parked the car and walked up the path of number ten.

And there was Hamish in the porch, coiled up comfortably on the mat, looking up at me with mild surprise as I hovered over him.

'Come on, lad,' I said. 'You've got more sense than we had. Why didn't we think of this before ?'

I deposited him on the passenger seat and as I drove away he hoisted his paws on to the dash and gazed out interestedly at the road unfolding in the headlights. Truly a phlegmatic little hound.

Outside Skeldale House I tucked him under my arm and was about to turn the handle of the front door when I paused. Tristan had notched up a long succession of successful pranks against me – fake telephone calls, the ghost in my bedroom and many others – and in fact, good friends as we were, he never neglected a chance to take the mickey out of me. In this situation, with the positions reversed, he would be merciless. I put my finger on the bell and leaned on it for several long seconds.

For some time there was neither sound nor movement from within and I pictured the cowering figure mustering his courage before marching to his doom. Then the light came on in the passage and as I peered expectantly through the glass a nose appeared round the far corner followed very gingerly by a wary eye. By degrees the full face inched into view and when Tristan recognized my grinning countenance he unleashed a cry of rage and bounded along the passage with upraised fist.

I really think that in his distraught state he would have attacked me, but the sight of Hamish banished all else. He grabbed the hairy creature and began to fondle him.

'Good little dog, nice little dog,' he crooned as he trotted

163

through to the sitting room. 'What a beautiful thing you are.' He laid him lovingly in the basket, and Hamish, after a 'heigh-ho, here we are again' glance around him, put his head along his side and promptly went to sleep.

Tristan fell limply into the armchair and gazed at me with glazed eyes.

'Well, we're saved, Jim,' he whispered. 'But I'll never be the same after tonight. I've run bloody miles and I've nearly lost my voice with shouting. I tell you I'm about knackered.'

I, too, was vastly relieved, and the nearness of catastrophe was brought home to us when Miss Westerman arrived within ten minutes.

'Oh, my darling!' she cried as Hamish leaped at her, mouth open, short tail wagging furiously. 'I've been so worried about you all day.'

She looked tentatively at the ear with its rows of buttons. 'Oh, it does look a lot better without that horrid swelling – and what a nice neat job you have made. Thank you, Mr Herriot, and thank you, too, young man.'

Tristan, who had staggered to his feet, bowed slightly as I showed the lady out.

'Bring him back in six weeks to have the stitches out,' I called to her as she left, then I rushed back into the room.

'Siegfried's just pulled up outside! You'd better look as if you've been working.'

He rushed to the bookshelves, pulled down Gaiger and Davis's *Bacteriology* and a notebook and dived into a chair. When his brother came in he was utterly engrossed.

Siegfried moved over to the fire and warmed his hands. He looked pink and mellow.

'I've just been speaking to Miss Westerman,' he said. 'She's really pleased. Well done, both of you.'

'Thank you,' I said, but Tristan was too busy to reply, scanning the pages anxiously and scribbling repeatedly in the notebook.

Siegfried walked behind the young man's chair and looked down at the open volume.

'Ah, yes, Clostridium septique,' he murmured, smiling indulgently. 'That's a good one to study. Keeps coming up in exams.'

He rested a hand briefly on his brother's shoulder. 'I'm glad to see you at work. You've been raking about too much lately and it's getting you down. A night at your books will have been good for you.'

He yawned, stretched, and made for the door. 'I'm off to bed. I'm rather sleepy.' He paused with his hand on the door. 'You know, Tristan, I quite envy you – there's nothing like a nice restful evening at home.'

18

When I was discharged from hospital I expected to be posted straight overseas and I wondered if I would be able to catch up with my old flight and my friends.

However, I learned with surprise that I had to go to a convalescent home for a fortnight before any further action could be taken. This was in Puddlestone, near Leominster – a lovely mansion house in acres of beautiful gardens. It was presided over by a delightful old matron with whom we fortunate airmen played sedate games of croquet or walked in the cool woods; it was easy to imagine there was no such thing as a war. Two weeks of this treatment left me feeling revitalized. It wouldn't be long, I felt, before I was back on the job.

From Puddlestone it was back to Manchester and Heaton Park again and this time it was strange to think that in all the great sprawl of huts and the crowding thousands of men in blue there wasn't a soul who knew me.

Except, of course, the Wing Commander who had sent me to hospital in the first place. I had an interview with him on my arrival and he came straight to the point.

'Herriot,' he said. 'I'm afraid you can't fly any more.'

'But . . . I've had the operation . . . I'm a lot better.'

'I know that, but you can no longer be classed as one hundred per cent fit. You have been officially downgraded and I'm sure you realize that pilots have to be grade one.'

'Yes ... of course.'

He glanced at the file in his hand. 'I see you are a veterinary surgeon. Mmm – this poses a problem. Normally when an aircrew is grounded he remusters on the ground staff, but yours is a reserved occupation. You really can't serve in any capacity but aircrew. Yes ... yes ... we'll have to see.'

It was all very impersonal and businesslike. Those few words coming from a man like him left no room for argument and they obliterated at a stroke every picture I had ever had of my future in the RAF.

I was fairly certain that if my flying days were over I would be discharged from the service and as I left the Wing Commander's office and walked slowly back to my hut at the other end of the park I pondered on my contribution to the war effort.

I hadn't fired a shot in anger. I had peeled mountains of potatoes, washed countless dishes, shovelled coke, mucked out pigs, marched for miles, drilled interminably, finally and magically learned to fly and now it was all for nothing. I passed the big dining hall and the RAF march blared out at me from the loud-speakers.

The familiar sound reminded me of so many experiences, so many friends, and suddenly I felt intensely lonely. I wanted somebody to talk to. It was a new sensation for me, and there, in those unlikely surroundings, I began to realize how much I used to enjoy chatting to the farmers during my veterinary calls.

It is one of the nicest things about country practice, but you have to keep your mind on the job at the same time or you could be in trouble. And at Mr Duggleby's I nearly landed in the biggest trouble of all. He was a smallholder who kept a few sows and reared the litters to pork weight in some ramshackle sheds behind the railway line outside Darrowby.

He was also a cricket fanatic, steeped in the lore and history of the game, and he would talk about it for hours on end. He never tired of it.

I was a willing listener because cricket has always fascinated me, even though I grew up in Scotland where it is little played. As I moved among the young pigs only part of my attention was focused on the little animals – most of me was out on the great green oval at Headingley with the Yorkshire heroes.

'By gaw, you should've seen Len Hutton on Saturday,' he breathed reverently. 'A hundred and eighty and never gave a chance. It was lovely to watch 'im.' He gave a fair imitation of the great man's cover drive.

'Yes, I can imagine it.' I nodded and smiled. 'You said these pigs were lame, Mr Duggleby?'

'Aye, noticed a few of 'em hoppin' about with a leg up this mornin'. And you know, Maurice Leyland was nearly as good. Not as classy as Len, tha knows, but by heck 'e can clump 'em.'

'Yes, he's a lion-hearted little player is Maurice,' I said. I reached down, grabbed a pig by the tail and thrust my thermometer into its rectum. 'Remember him and Eddie Paynter in the test match against Australia?'

He gave a dreamy smile. 'Remember it? By gaw, that's summat I'll never forget. What a day that was.'

I withdrew the thermometer. 'This little chap's got a temperature of a hundred and five. Must be some infection somewhere – maybe a touch of joint ill.' I felt my way along the small pink limbs. 'And yet it's funny, the joints aren't swollen.'

'Ah reckon Bill Bowes'll skittle Somerset out when they start their innings today. This wicket's just to 'is liking.'

'Yes, he's a great bowler, isn't he?' I said. 'I love watching a good fast bowler. I suppose you'll have seen them all – Larwood, Voce, G. O. Allen and the rest?'

'Aye, that I have. I could go on all day about those men.'

I caught another of the lame pigs and examined it. 'This is rather strange, Mr Duggleby. About half the pigs in this pen seem to be lame but there's nothing to see.'

'Aye well, happen it's like you said – joint ill. You can give 'em a jab for that, can't you? And while you're doin' it I'll tell you of the time I saw Wilfred Rhodes take eight wickets in an afternoon.'

I filled a syringe. 'Right, we'd better give them all a shot. Have you got a marking pencil there?'

The farmer nodded and lifted one of the little animals which promptly unleashed a protesting scream. 'There was never anybody like awd Wilfred,' he shouted above the noise. 'It was about half past two and the wicket had had a shower of rain on it when t'skipper threw 'im the ball.'

I smile and raised my syringe. It passed the time so pleasantly listening to these reminiscences. Well content, I was about to plunge the needle into the pink thigh when one of the pigs began to nibble at the heel of my wellington. I looked down at a ring of the little creatures all looking up at me, alarmed by the shrill screeches of their friend.

My mind was still with Wilfred Rhodes when I noticed what looked like a small white knob on one of the uptilted snouts. And there was another on that one – and that one . . . I had been unable to see their faces until now because they had been trying to run away from me, but a warning bell clanged suddenly in my head.

I reached down and seized a pig, and as I squeezed the swelling on the snout a cold wind blew through me, scattering the gentle vision of cricket and sunshine and green grass. It wasn't a knob, it was a vesicle, a delicate blister which ruptured easily on pressure.

I could feel my arms shaking as I turned the piglet up and began to examine the tiny cloven feet. There were more vesicles there, flatter and more diffuse, but telling the same dread story.

Dry-mouthed, I lifted two other pigs. They were just the same. As I turned to the farmer I felt bowed down by a crushing weight of pity, almost of guilt. He was still smiling eagerly, anxious to get on with his tale, and I was about to give him the worst news a veterinary surgeon can give a stockman.

'Mr Duggleby,' I said. 'I'm afraid I'll have to telephone the Ministry of Agriculture.'

'The Ministry . . . ? What for ?'

'To tell them I have a case of suspected Foot and Mouth Disease.'

'Foot and Mouth ? Never !'

'Yes, I'm terribly sorry.'

'Are you sure ?'

'It's not up to me to be definite about it, Mr Duggleby. One of the Ministry officers will have to do that – I must phone them right away.'

It was an unlikely place to find a telephone but Mr Duggleby ran a little coal delivery round on the side. I was quickly through to the Ministry and I spoke to Neville Craggs, one of the full-time officers.

He groaned. 'Sounds awfully like it, Jim. Anyway, stay put till I see you.'

In the farm kitchen Mr Duggleby looked at me inquiringly. 'What now?'

'You'll just have to put up with me for a bit,' I said. 'I can't leave till I get the verdict.'

He was silent for a moment. 'What happens if it's what you think?'

'I'm afraid your pigs will have to be slaughtered.'

'Every one of 'em?'

'That is the law – I'm sorry. But you'll get compensation.'

He scratched his head. 'But they can get better. Why do you have to kill 'em all?'

'You're quite right.' I shrugged. 'Many animals do recover, but Foot and Mouth is fiercely infectious. While you were treating them it would have spread to neighbouring farms, then all over the country.'

'Aye, but look at the expense. Slaughtering must cost thousands o' pounds.'

'I agree, but it would cost a lot more the other way. Apart from the animals that die, just think of the loss of milk, loss of flesh in cows, pigs and sheep. It would come to millions every year. It's lucky Britain is an island.'

'Reckon you'll be right.' He felt for his pipe. 'And you're pretty sure I've got it?'

'Yes.'

'Aye well,' he murmured. 'These things 'appen.'

The old Yorkshire words. I had heard them so often under circumstances which would make most city folk, including myself, beat their heads against a wall. Mr Duggleby's smallholding would soon be a silent place of death, but he just chewed his pipe and said, 'These things 'appen.'

It didn't take the Ministry long to make up their minds. The source of the infection was almost certainly some imported meat which Mr Duggleby hadn't boiled properly with his swill. The disease was confirmed and a fifteen-mile radius standstill order was imposed. I disinfected myself and my car and went home. I undressed, my clothes were taken away for fumigation and I climbed into a hot antiseptic bath.

Lying there in the steam, I pondered on what might have been. If I had failed to spot the disease I would have gone merrily on my way, spreading destruction and havoc. I always washed my boots before leaving a farm, but how about those little pigs nibbling round the hem of my long coat, how about my syringe, even my thermometer? My next call was to have been to Terence Bailey's pedigree herd of dairy shorthorns – two hundred peerless cows, a strain built up over generations. Foreigners came from all over the world to buy them and I could have been the cause of their annihilation.

And then there was Mr Duggleby himself. I could picture him rattling around the farms in his coal wagon. He would have done his bit of spreading, too. And like as not he would have taken a few store pigs to the auction mart this week, sending the deadly contagion all over Yorkshire and beyond. It was easy to see how a major outbreak could have started – a disaster of national importance costing millions.

If I hadn't been sweating already I would have started now at the very thought of it. I would have joined the unhappy band of practitioners who had missed Foot and Mouth.

I knew of some of these people and my heart bled for them. It could happen so easily. Busy men trying to examine kicking, struggling animals in dark buildings with perhaps part of their mind on the list of calls ahead. And the other hazards – the total unexpectedness, the atypical case, various distractions. My distraction had been cricket and it had nearly caused my downfall. But I had escaped and, huddling lower in the hot water, I said a silent prayer of thanks.

Later, with a complete change of clothes and instruments, I continued on my rounds and as I stood in Terence Bailey's long byre I realized my luck again. The long rows of beautiful animals, meticulously groomed, firm high udders pushing between their hocks, delicate heads, fine legs deep in straw; they were a picture of bovine perfection and quite irreplaceable.

Once Foot and Mouth is confirmed in a district there is a tense period of waiting. Farmers, veterinary surgeons and most of all, Ministry officials are on the rack, wondering if there has been any dissemination before diagnosis, bracing themselves against the telephone message which could herald the raging spread which they dreaded and which would tear their lives apart.

To the city dwellers a big Foot and Mouth outbreak is something remote which they read about in the newspapers. To the country folk it means the transformation of the quiet farms and fields into charnel houses and funeral pyres. It means heartbreak and ruin.

We waited in Darrowby. And as the days passed and no frightening news of lame or salivating animals came over the wires it seemed that the Duggleby episode was what we hoped – an isolated case caused by a few shreds of imported meat.

I almost bathed in disinfectant on every farm, sloshing a strong solution of Lysol over my boots and protective clothing so that my car reeked of the stuff and I caused wrinkled noses when I entered a shop, the post office, the bank.

After nearly two weeks I had begun to feel reasonably safe, but when I had a call from the famous Bailey farm I felt a twinge of apprehension.

It was Terence Bailey himself. 'Will you come and see one of my cows, Mr Herriot. She's got blisters on one of her teats.'

'Blisters!' My heart went bump. 'Is she slavering, is she lame?'

'Nay, nay, she just has these nasty blisters. Seem to have fluid in them.'

I was breathless as I put down the receiver. One nasty blister would be enough. It sometimes started like that in cows. I almost ran out to my car and on the journey my mind beat about like a trapped bird.

Bailey's was the farm I had visited straight from Duggleby's. Could I possibly have carried it there? But the change of clothes, the bath, the fresh thermometer and instruments. What more could I do? How about my car wheels? Well, I had disinfected them, too – I couldn't possibly be blamed, but ... but ...

It was Mr Bailey's wife who met me.

'I noticed this cow when I was milking this morning, Mr Herriot.' The herd was still hand-milked and in the hardworking family tradition Mrs Bailey did her stint night and morning with her husband and the farm men.

'As soon as I got hold of the teats I could see the cow was uneasy,' she continued. 'Then I saw there was a lot of little blisters and one big one. I managed to milk her and most of the little blisters burst, but the big one's still there.'

I bent and peered anxiously at the udder. It was as she said – lots of small ruptured vesicles and one large one, intact and fluctuating. It was all horribly evocative and without speaking I moved along, grasped the cow's nose and pulled her head round. I prised the mouth open and stared desperately at lips, cheek and dental pad. I think I would have fainted if I had found anything in there but it was all clean and normal.

I lifted each forefoot in turn and scrubbed out the clefts with soap and water – nothing. I tied a rope round the hind leg, threw it over a beam and with the help of one of the men pulled the foot up. More scrubbing and searching without success then the same with the other hind foot. When I finished I was perspiring but no further forward.

I took the temperature and found it slightly elevated, then I walked up and down the byre.

'Is there any trouble among these other cows?' I asked.

Mrs Bailey shook her head. 'No, there's just this one.' She was a good-looking woman in her thirties with the red, roughened complexion of the outdoor worker. 'What do you think it is?'

I didn't dare tell her. I had a cow with vesicles on the teats right in the middle of a district under Foot and Mouth restrictions. I just couldn't take a chance. I had to bring the Ministry in.

Even then I was unable to speak the dread words. All I could say was, 'Can I use your phone, please?'

She looked surprised, but smiled quickly. 'Yes, of course. Come into the house.'

As I walked down the byre I looked again at the beautiful cows and then beyond, at the fold yard where I could see the young heifers and the tiny calves in their pens. All of them carrying the Bailey blood which had been produced and perfected by generations of careful breeding and selection. But a humane killer is no respecter of such things and if my fears were realized a quick series of bang-bangs would wipe out all this in an hour or two.

We went into the farm kitchen and Mrs Bailey pointed to the door at the far end.

'The phone's through there in the front room,' she said.

I kicked off my wellingtons and was padding across the floor in my stockinged feet when I almost fell over Giles, the lusty one-year-old baby of the family, as he waddled across my path. I bent to ease him out of the way and he looked up at me with an enormous cheesy grin.

His mother laughed. 'Just look at him. Full of the devil, and he's had such a painful arm since his smallpox vaccination.'

'Poor lad,' I said absently, patting his head as I opened the door, my mind already busy with the uncomfortable conversation ahead. I had taken a few strides over the carpet beyond, when I halted abruptly.

I turned and looked back into the kitchen. 'Did you say small-pox vaccination ?'

'Yes, all our other children have been done when they were his age but they've never reacted like this. I've had to change his dressing every day.'

'You changed his dressing . . . and you milked that cow . . . ?'

'Yes, that's right.'

A great light beamed suddenly, spilling sunshine into my dark troubled world. I returned to the kitchen and closed the door behind me.

Mrs Bailey looked at me for a moment in silence, then she spoke hesitantly. 'Aren't you going to use the phone ?'

'No . . . no . . .' I replied. 'I've changed my mind.'

'I see.' She raised her eyebrows and seemed at a loss for words. Then she smiled and lifted the kettle. 'Well, maybe you'll have a cup of tea, then ?'

'Thank you, that would be lovely.' I sank happily on to one of the hard wooden chairs.

Mrs Bailey put the kettle on and turned to me. 'By the way, you've never told me what's wrong with that cow.'

'Oh yes, of course, I'm sorry,' I said airily as though I'd just forgotten to mention it. 'She's got cow pox. In fact you gave it to her.'

'I gave it . . . ? What do you mean ?'

'Well, the vaccine they use for babies is made from the cow pox virus. You carried it on your hands from the baby to the cow.' I smiled, enjoying my big moment.

Her mouth fell open slightly, then she began to giggle. 'Oh dear, I don't know what my husband's going to say. I've never heard of anything like that.' She wiggled her fingers in front of her eyes. 'And I'm always so careful, too. But I've been a bit harassed with the poor little chap's arm.'

'Oh well, it isn't serious,' I said. 'I've got some ointment in the car which will cure it quite quickly.'

I sipped my tea and watched Giles's activities. In a short time he had spread chaos throughout the kitchen and at the moment was busily engaged in removing all the contents of a cupboard in the corner. Bent double, small bottom out-thrust, he hurled pans, lids, brushes behind him with intense dedication till the cupboard was empty. Then, as he looked around for further employment, he spotted me and tacked towards me on straddled legs.

My stocking-clad toes seemed to fascinate him and as I wiggled them at him he grasped at them with fat little hands. When he had finally trapped my big toe he looked up at me with his huge grin in which four tiny teeth glittered.

I smiled back at him with sincere affection as the relief flowed through me. It wasn't just that I was grateful to him – I really liked him. I still like Giles today. He is one of my clients, a burly farmer with a family of his own, a deep love and knowledge of pedigree cows and the same big grin, except that there are a few more teeth in it.

But he'll never know how near his smallpox vaccination came to giving me heart failure.

19

I looked around me at the heap of boots, the piled mounds of shirts, the rows of empty shelves and pigeon holes. I was employed in the stores at Heaton Park, living proof that the RAF was finding me something of a problem.

The big war machine was rumbling along pretty smoothly by this time, turning out pilots, navigators, air-gunners in a steady stream and slotting them into different jobs if they failed to make the grade. It ticked over like a well-oiled engine as long as nothing disturbed the rhythm.

I was like a speck of sand in the works, and I could tell from various interviews that I had caused the administrators a certain amount of puzzlement. I don't suppose Mr Churchill was losing any sleep over me but since I wasn't allowed to fly and was ineligible for the ground staff I was obviously a bit of a nuisance. Nobody seemed to have come across a grounded vet before.

Of course it was inevitable that I would be sent back to my practice, but I could see that it was going to take some time for the RAF to regurgitate me into civil life. Apparently I had to go through the motions even though some of them were meaningless.

One of the interviews was with three officers. They were very nice and they sat behind a table, beaming, friendly, reassuring. Their task, apparently, was to find out what ground staff job might suit me. I think they were probably psychologists and they asked me all kinds of questions, nodding and smiling kindly all the time.

'Well now, Herriot,' the middle officer said. 'We are going to put you through a series of aptitude tests. It will last two days, starting tomorrow, and by the end of it I think we'll know all about you.' He laughed. 'It's nothing to worry about. You might rather enjoy it.'

I did enjoy it, in fact. I filled up great long sheets with my answers, I drew diagrams, fitted odd-shaped pieces of wood into holes. It was fun.

I had to wait another two days before I was called before the tribunal again. The three were if anything more charming than before and I seemed to sense an air of subdued excitement about them this time. They were all smiling broadly as the middle one spoke.

'Herriot, we have really found out something about you,' he said.

'You have?'

'Yes, indeed. We have found that you have an outstanding mechanical aptitude.'

I stared at him. This was a facer, because if ever there was a mechanical idiot that man is J. Herriot. I have a loathing for engines, wheels, pistons, cylinders, cogs. I can't mend anything and if a garage mechanic tries to explain something to me I just can't take it in.

I told the officers this and the three smiles became rather fixed.

'But surely,' said the one on the left, 'you drive a car in the course of your professional work ?'

'Yes, sir, I do. I've driven one for years, but I still don't know how it works and if I break down I have to scream for help.'

'I see, I see.' The smiles were very thin now and the three heads came together for a whispered consultation.

Finally the middle one leaned across the table.

'Tell you what, Herriot. How would you like to be a meteorologist ?'

'Fine,' I replied.

I sympathized with them, because they were obviously kind men, but I've never had any faith in aptitude tests since then.

Of course there was never the slightest chance of my becoming a meteorologist and I suppose that's how I landed in the stores. It was one of the bizarre periods of my life, mercifully brief but vivid. They had told me to report to Corporal Weekes at the stores hut and I made my way through the maze of roads of a Heaton Park populated by strangers.

Corporal Weekes was fat and he gave me a quick look over with crafty eyes.

'Herriot, eh ? Well you can make yourself useful around 'ere. Not much to do, really. This ain't a main stores – we deal mainly wiv laundry and boot repairs.'

As he spoke a fair-haired young man came in.

'AC2 Morgan, Corporal,' he said. 'Come for my boots. They've been re-soled.'

Weekes jerked his head and I had my first sight of the boot mountain. 'They're in there. They'll be labelled.'

The young man looked surprised but he came round behind the counter and began to delve among the hundreds of identical black objects. It took him nearly an hour to find his own pair during which the corporal puffed at cigarettes with a total lack of interest. When the boots were finally unearthed he wordlessly ticked off the name on a long list.

'This is the sort of thing you'll be doin', he said to me. 'Nothin' to it.'

He wasn't exaggerating. There was nothing to life in those stores. It took me only a day or two to realize the sweet existence Weekes had carved out for himself. Store-bashing is an honourable trade but not the way he did it. The innumerable compartments, niches and alcoves around the big hut were all marked with letters or numbers and there is no doubt the incoming boots and shirts should have been tucked away in order for easy recovery. But that would have involved work and the corporal was clearly averse to that.

When the boots came in they were tipped out in the middle of the floor and the string-tied packages of laundry were stacked, shirts-uppermost where they formed a blue tumulus reaching almost to the roof.

After three days I could stand it no longer.

'Look,' I said. 'It would pass the time if I had something to do. Do you mind if I start putting all this stuff on the shelves? It would be a lot easier to hand out.'

Weekes continued to study his magazine – he was a big reader – and at first I thought he hadn't heard me. Then he tongued his cigarette to the corner of his mouth and glanced at me through the smoke.

'Now just get this through your 'ead, mate,' he drawled. 'If I want any — thing doin' I'll — well tell you. I'm the boss in 'ere and I give the — orders, awright ?' He resumed his perusal of the magazine.

I subsided in my chair. Clearly I had offended my overseer and I would have to leave things as they were.

But overseer is a misnomer for Weekes because on the following day, after a final brain-washing that the procedure must remain unchanged, he disappeared and except for a few minutes each morning he left me on my own. I had nothing to do but sit there behind the wooden counter, ticking off the comings and going of the boots and shirts and I had the feeling that I was only one of many displaced persons who had fallen under his thrall.

I found it acutely embarrassing to watch the lads scrabbling for their belongings and the strongest impression left with me was of the infinite tolerance of the British race. Since I was in

177

charge they thought I was responsible for the whole system but despite the fact that I was of lowly rank nobody attacked me physically. Most of them muttered and grumbled as they searched and one large chap came over to the counter and said, 'You should be filing away these boots in their proper order instead of sitting there on your arse, you lazy sod!' But he didn't punch me on the nose and I marvelled at it.

But still, the knowledge that great numbers of decent young men shared his opinion was uncomfortable and I found I was developing a permanently ingratiating smile.

The only time I came very near to being lynched was when a mob suddenly appeared one afternoon. An unexpected leave pass had been granted and there were hundreds of men milling around on the tarmac and grass outside the stores. They wanted their laundry – and quick, because they had trains to catch.

For a moment panic seized me. I couldn't let them all inside to fight for their shirts. Then inspiration came. I grabbed an armful of the flat packets from the table and shouted the name on the label.

'Walters!' And from somewhere among the surging heads an eager voice replied, 'Here!'

I located the source, held the packet between thumb and finger and with a back-hand flick sent it skimming over the crowd.

'Reilly!'

'Here!'

'McDonald!'

'Here!'

'Gibson!'

'Here!'

I was getting quite skilful at it, propelling the blue oblongs unerringly towards their owners, but it was a slow method of distribution. Also, there were occasional disasters when the strings broke in mid-air, sending a shower of collars on the upturned faces. Sometimes the shirts themselves burst free from their wrapping and plunged to earth.

It wasn't long before the voices had turned from eager to angry. As my projectiles planed and glided, volleys of abuse came back at me.

'You've made me miss my train, you useless bugger!'

'Bloody skiver, you want locking up!'

Much of it was in stronger language which I would rather not record here, but I have a particularly vivid memory of one young man scraping up his laundry from the dusty ground and approaching me with rapid strides. He pushed his face to within inches of mine. Despite the rage which disfigured it I could see it was a gentle, good-natured face. He looked a well-bred lad, the type who didn't even swear, but as he stared into my eyes his lips trembled and his cheeks twitched.

'This is a . . .' he stammered. 'This is a . . . a *bastard* system!' He spat the words out and strode away.

I agreed entirely with him, of course, but continued to hurl the packets doggedly while somewhere in the back of my mind a little voice kept inquiring how James Herriot, Member of the Royal College of Veterinary Surgeons and trainee pilot, had ever got into this.

After half an hour there was no appreciable dimunution in the size of the multitude and I began to be aware of an increasing restlessness among the medley of waiting faces.

Suddenly there was a concerted movement and the packed mass of men surged at me in a great wave. I shrank back, clutching an armful of shirts, quite certain that this was when they rushed me and beat me up, but my fears were groundless. All they wanted was a speedier delivery and about a dozen of them swept past me behind the counter and began to follow my example.

Whereas there had been only a single missile winging over the heads the sky was now dark with the flying objects. Mid-air collisions were frequent. Collars sprayed, handkerchiefs fluttered, underpants parachuted gracefully, but after an unbearably long period of chaos the last airman had picked up his scattered laundry, given me a disgusted glance and departed.

I was left alone in the hut with the sad knowledge that my prestige was very low and the equally sad conviction that the RAF still did not know what do do with me.

20

Occasionally my period in limbo was relieved when I was allowed out of camp into the city of Manchester. And I suppose it was the fact that I was a new-fangled parent that made me look at the various prams in the streets. Mostly the prams were pushed by women, but now and then I saw a man doing the job.

I suppose it isn't unusual to see a man pushing a pram in a town, but on a lonely moorland road the sight merits a second glance. Especially when the pram contains a large dog.

That was what I saw in the hills above Darrowby one morning and I slowed down as I drove past. I had noticed the strange combination before – on several occasions over the last few weeks – and it was clear that man and dog had recently moved into the district.

As the car drew abreast of him the man turned, smiled and raised his hand. It was a smile of rare sweetness in a very brown face. A forty-year-old face, I thought, above a brown neck which bore neither collar nor tie, and a faded striped shirt lying open over a bare chest despite the coldness of the day.

I couldn't help wondering who or what he was. The outfit of scuffed suede golf jacket, corduroy trousers and sturdy boots didn't give much clue. Some people might have put him down as an ordinary tramp, but there was a businesslike energetic look about him which didn't fit the term.

I wound the window down and the thin wind of a Yorkshire March bit at my cheeks.

'Nippy this morning,' I said.

The man seemed surprised. 'Aye,' he replied after a moment. 'Aye, reckon it is.'

I looked at the pram, ancient and rusty, and at the big animal sitting upright inside it. He was a lurcher, a cross-bred greyhound, and he gazed back at me with unruffled dignity.

'Nice dog,' I said.

'Aye, that's Jake.' The man smiled again, showing good regular teeth. 'He's a grand 'un.'

I waved and drove on. In the mirror I could see the compact figure stepping out briskly, head up, shoulders squared, and, rising like a statue from the middle of the pram, the huge brindled form of Jake.

I didn't have to wait long to meet the unlikely pair again. I was examining a carthorse's teeth in a farmyard when on the hillside beyond the stable I saw a figure kneeling by a dry stone wall. And by his side, a pram and a big dog sitting patiently on the grass.

'Hey, just a minute.' I pointed at the hill. 'Who is that?'

The farmer laughed. 'That's Roddy Travers. D'you ken 'im?'

'No, no I don't. I had a word with him on the road the other day, that's all.'

'Aye, on the road.' He nodded knowingly. 'That's where you'd see Roddy, right enough.'

'But what is he? Where does he come from?'

'He comes from somewhere in Yorkshire, but ah don't rightly know where and ah don't think anybody else does. But I'll tell you this – he can turn 'is hand to anything.'

'Yes,' I said, watching the man expertly laying the flat slabs of stone as he repaired a gap in the wall. 'There's not many can do what he's doing now.'

'That's true. Wallin' is a skilled job and it's dying out, but Roddy's a dab hand at it. But he can do owt – hedgin', ditchin', lookin' after stock, it's all the same to him.'

I lifted the tooth rasp and began to rub a few sharp corners off the horse's molars. 'And how long will he stay here?'

'Oh, when he's finished that wall he'll be off. Ah could do with 'im stoppin' around for a bit but he never stays in one place for long.'

'But hasn't he got a home anywhere?'

'Nay, nay.' The farmer laughed again. 'Roddy's got nowt. All 'e has in the world is in that there pram.'

Over the next weeks as the harsh spring began to soften and the sunshine brought a bright speckle of primroses on to the grassy banks I saw Roddy quite often, sometimes on the road, occasionally wielding a spade busily on the ditches around the fields. Jake was always there, either loping by his side or watching him at work. But we didn't actually meet again till I was inoculating Mr Pawson's sheep for pulpy kidney.

There were three hundred to do and they drove them in batches into a small pen where Roddy caught and held them for me. And I could see he was an expert at this, too. The wild hill sheep whipped past him like bullets but he seized their fleece effortlessly, sometimes in mid-air, and held the foreleg up to expose that bare clean area of skin behind the elbow that nature seemed to provide for the veterinary surgeon's needle.

Outside, on the windy slopes the big lurcher sat upright in typical pose, looking with mild interest at the farm dogs prowling intently around the pens, but not interfering in any way.

'You've got him well trained,' I said.

Roddy smiled. 'Yes, ye'll never find Jake dashin' about, annoyin' people. He knows 'e has to sit there till I'm finished and there he'll sit.'

'And quite happy to do so, by the look of him.' I glanced again at the dog, a picture of contentment. 'He must live a wonderful life, travelling everywhere with you.'

'You're right there,' Mr Pawson broke in as he ushered another bunch of sheep into the pen. 'He hasn't a care in t'world, just like his master.'

Roddy didn't say anything, but as the sheep ran in he straightened up and took a long steady breath. He had been working hard and a little trickle of sweat ran down the side of his forehead but as he gazed over the wide sweep of moor and fell I could read utter serenity in his face. After a few moments he spoke.

'I reckon that's true. We haven't much to worry us, Jake and me.'

Mr Pawson grinned mischievously. 'By gaw, Roddy, you never spoke a truer word. No wife, no kids, no life insurance, no overdraft at t'bank – you must have a right peaceful existence.'

'Ah suppose so,' Roddy said. 'But then ah've no money either.'

The farmer gave him a quizzical look. 'Aye, how about that, then? Wouldn't you feel a bit more secure, like, if you had a bit o' brass put by?'

'Nay, nay. Ye can't take it with you and any road, as long as a man can pay 'is way, he's got enough.'

There was nothing original about the words, but they have

stayed with me all my life because they came from his lips and were spoken with such profound assurance.

When I had finished the inoculations and the ewes were turned out to trot back happily over the open fields I turned to Roddy. 'Well, thanks very much. It makes my job a lot quicker when I have a good catcher like you.' I pulled out a packet of Gold Flake. 'Will you have a cigarette?'

'No, thank ye, Mr Herriot. I don't smoke.'

'You don't?'

'No – don't drink either.' He gave me his gentle smile and again I had the impression of physical and mental purity. No drinking, no smoking, a life of constant movement in the open air without material possessions or ambitions – it all showed in the unclouded eyes, the fresh skin and the hard muscular frame. He wasn't very big but he looked indestructible.

'C'mon, Jake, it's dinnertime,' he said and the big lurcher bounded around him in delight. I went over and spoke to the dog and he responded with tremendous body-swaying wags, his handsome face looking up at me, full of friendliness.

I stroked the long pointed head and tickled the ears. 'He's a beauty, Roddy – a grand 'un, as you said.'

I walked to the house to wash my hands and before I went inside I glanced back at the two of them. They were sitting in the shelter of a wall and Roddy was laying out a thermos flask and a parcel of food while Jake watched eagerly. The hard bright sunshine beat on them as the wind whistled over the top of the wall. They looked supremely comfortable and at peace.

'He's independent, you see,' the farmer's wife said as I stood at the kitchen sink. 'He's welcome to come in for a bit o' dinner but he'd rather stay outside with his dog.'

I nodded. 'Where does he sleep when he's going round the farms like this?'

'Oh, anywhere,' she replied. 'In hay barns or granaries or sometimes out in the open, but when he's with us he sleeps upstairs in one of our rooms. Ah know for a fact any of the farmers would be willin' to have him in the house because he allus keeps himself spotless clean.'

'I see.' I pulled the towel from behind the door. 'He's quite a character, isn't he?'

She smiled ruminatively. 'Aye, he certainly is. Just him and his dog!' She lifted a fragrant dishful of hot roast ham from the oven and set it on the table. 'But I'll tell you this. The feller's all right. Everybody likes Roddy Travers – he's a very nice man.'

Roddy stayed around the Darrowby district throughout the summer and I grew used to the sight of him on the farms or pushing his pram along the roads. When it was raining he wore a tattered over-long gaberdine coat, but at other times it was always the golf jacket and corduroys. I don't know where he had accumulated his wardrobe. It was a safe bet he had never been on a golf course in his life and it was just another of the little mysteries about him.

I saw him early one morning on a hill path in early October. It had been a night of iron frost and the tussocky pastures beyond the walls were held in a pitiless white grip with every blade of grass stiffly ensheathed in rime.

I was muffled to the eyes and had been beating my gloved fingers against my knees to thaw them out, but when I pulled up and wound down the window the first thing I saw was the bare chest under the collarless unbuttoned shirt.

'Mornin', Mr Herriot,' he said. 'Ah'm glad I've seen ye.' He paused and gave me his tranquil smile. 'There's a job along t'road for a couple of weeks, then I'm movin' on.'

'I see.' I knew enough about him now not to ask where he was going. Instead I looked down at Jake who was sniffling the herbage. 'I see he's walking this morning.'

Roddy laughed. 'Yes, sometimes 'e likes to walk, sometimes 'e likes to ride. He pleases 'imself.'

'Right, Roddy,' I said. 'No doubt we'll meet again. All the best to you.'

He waved and set off jauntily over the icebound road and I felt that a little vein of richness had gone from my life.

But I was wrong. That same evening about eight o'clock the front door bell rang. I answered it and found Roddy on the front doorsteps. Behind him, just visible in the frosty darkness, stood the ubiquitous pram.

'I want you to look at me dog, Mr Herriot,' he said.

'Why, what's the trouble ?'

'Ah don't rightly know. He's havin' sort of . . . faintin' fits.'

'Fainting fits? That doesn't sound like Jake. Where is he, anyway?'

He pointed behind him 'In t'pram, under t'cover.'

'All right.' I threw the door wide. 'Bring him in.'

Roddy adroitly manhandled the rusty old vehicle up the steps and pushed it, squeaking and rattling, along the passage to the consulting room. There, under the bright lights he snapped back the fasteners and threw off the cover to reveal Jake stretched beneath.

His head was pillowed on the familiar gaberdine coat and around him lay his master's worldly goods; a string-tied bundle of spare shirt and socks, a packet of tea, a thermos, knife and spoon and an ex-army haversack.

The big dog looked up at me with terrified eyes and as I patted him I could feel his whole frame quivering.

'Let him lie there a minute, Roddy,' I said. 'And tell me exactly what you've seen.'

He rubbed his palms together and his fingers trembled. 'Well, it only started this afternoon. He was right as rain, larkin' about on the grass, then he went into a sort o' fit.'

'How do you mean?'

'Just kind of seized up and toppled over on 'is side. He lay there for a bit, gaspin' and slaverin'. Ah'll tell ye, I thought he was a goner.' His eyes widened and a corner of his mouth twitched at the memory.

'How long did that last?'

'Nobbut a few seconds. Then he got up and you'd say there was nowt wrong with 'im.'

'But he did it again?'

'Aye, time and time again. Drove me near daft. But in between 'e was normal. Normal, Mr Herriot!'

It sounded ominously like the onset of epilepsy. 'How old is he?' I asked.

'Five gone last February.'

Ah well, it was a bit old for that. I reached for a stethoscope and auscultated the heart. I listened intently but heard only the racing beat of a frightened animal. There was no abnormality. My thermometer showed no rise in temperature.

'Let's have him on the table, Roddy. You take the back end.'

The big animal was limp in our arms as we hoisted him on to the smooth surface, but after lying there for a moment he looked timidly around him then sat up with a slow and careful movement. As we watched he reached out and licked his master's face while his tail flickered between his legs.

'Look at that!' the man exclaimed. 'He's all right again. You'd think he didn't ail a thing.'

And indeed Jake was recovering his confidence rapidly. He peered tentatively at the floor a few times then suddenly jumped down, trotted to his master and put his paws against his chest.

I looked at the dog standing there, tail wagging furiously. 'Well, that's a relief, anyway. I didn't like the look of him just then, but whatever's been troubling him seems to have righted itself. I'll . . .'

My happy flow was cut off. I stared at the lurcher. His forelegs were on the floor again and his mouth was gaping as he fought for breath. Frantically he gasped and retched then he blundered across the floor, collided with the pram wheels and fell on his side.

'What the hell . . .! Quick, get him up again!' I grabbed the animal round the middle and we lifted him back on to the table.

I watched in disbelief as the huge form lay there. There was no fight for breath now – he wasn't breathing at all, he was unconscious. I pushed my fingers inside his thigh and felt the pulse. It was still going, rapid and feeble, but yet he didn't breathe.

He could die any moment and I stood there helpless, all my scientific training useless. Finally my frustration burst from me and I struck the dog on the ribs with the flat of my hand.

'Jake!' I yelled. 'Jake, what's the matter with you ?'

As though in reply, the lurcher immediately started to take great wheezing breaths, his eyelids twitched back to consciousness and he began to look about him. But he was still mortally afraid and he lay prone as I gently stroked his head.

There was a long silence while the animal's terror slowly subsided, then he sat up on the table and regarded us placidly.

'There you are,' Roddy said softly. 'Same thing again. Ah can't reckon it up and ah thought ah knew summat about dogs.'

I didn't say anything. I couldn't reckon it up either, and I was supposed to be a veterinary surgeon.

I spoke at last. 'Roddy, that wasn't a fit. He was choking. Something was interfering with his air flow.' I took my hand torch from my breast pocket. 'I'm going to have a look at his throat.'

I pushed Jake's jaws apart, depressed his tongue with a forefinger and shone the light into the depths. He was the kind of good-natured dog who offered no resistance as I prodded around, but despite my floodlit view of the pharynx I could find nothing wrong. I had been hoping desperately to come across a bit of bone stuck there somewhere but I ranged feverishly over pink tongue, healthy tonsils and gleaming molars without success. Everything looked perfect.

I was tilting his head a little further when I felt him stiffen and heard Roddy's cry.

'He's goin' again!'

And he was, too. I stared in horror as the brindled body slid away from me and lay prostrate once more on the table. And again the mouth strained wide and froth bubbled round the lips. As before, the breathing had stopped and the rib cage was motionless. As the seconds ticked away I beat on the chest with my hand but it didn't work this time. I pulled the lower eyelid down from the staring orb – the conjunctiva was blue, Jake hadn't long to live. The tragedy of the thing bore down on me. This wasn't just a dog, he was this man's family and I was watching him die.

It was at that moment that I heard the faint sound. It was a strangled cough which barely stirred the dog's lips.

'Damn it!' I shouted. 'He *is* choking. There must be something down there.'

Again I seized the head and pushed my torch into the mouth and I shall always be thankful that at that very instant the dog coughed again, opening the cartilages of the larynx and giving me a glimpse of the cause of all the trouble. There, beyond the drooping epiglottis I saw for a fleeting moment a smooth round object no bigger than a pea.

'I think it's a pebble,' I gasped. 'Right inside his larynx.'

'You mean, in 'is Adam's apple?'

'That's right, and it's acting like a ball valve, blocking his wind-pipe every now and then.' I shook the dog's head. 'You see, look, I've dislodged it for the moment. He's coming round again.'

Once more Jake was reviving and breathing steadily.

Roddy ran his hand over the head, along the back and down the great muscles of the hind limbs. 'But . . . but . . . it'll happen again, won't it ?'

I nodded. 'I'm afraid so.'

'And one of these times it isn't goin' to shift and that'll be the end of 'im ?' He had gone very pale.

'That's about it, Roddy, I'll have to get that pebble out.'

'But how . . . ?'

'Cut into the larynx. And right now – it's the only way.'

'All right.' He swallowed. 'Let's get on. I don't think ah could stand it if he went down again.'

I knew what he meant. My knees had begun to shake, and I had a strong conviction that if Jake collapsed once more then so would I.

I seized a pair of scissors and clipped away the hair from the ventral surface of the larynx. I dared not use a general anaesthetic and infiltrated the area with local before swabbing with antisep-tic. Mercifully there was a freshly boiled set of instruments lying in the sterilizer and I lifted out the tray and set it on the trolley by the side of the table.

'Hold his head steady,' I said hoarsely, and gripped a scalpel.

I cut down through skin, fascia and the thin layers of the sterno-hyoid and omo-hyoid muscles till the ventral surface of the larynx was revealed. This was something I had never done to a live dog before, but desperation abolished any hesitancy and it took me only another few seconds to incise the thin membrane and peer into the interior.

And there it was. A pebble right enough – grey and glistening and tiny, but big enough to kill.

I had to fish it out quickly and cleanly without pushing it into the trachea. I leaned back and rummaged in the tray till I found some broad-bladed forceps, then I poised them over the wound. Great surgeons' hands, I felt sure, didn't shake like this, nor did such men pant as I was doing. But I clenched my teeth, introduced the forceps and my hand magically steadied as I clamped them over the pebble.

I stopped panting, too. In fact I didn't breathe at all as I bore the shining little object slowly and tenderly through the opening and dropped it with a gentle rat-tat on the table.

'Is that it?' asked Roddy, almost in a whisper.

'That's it.' I reached for needle and suture silk. 'All is well now.'

The stitching took only a few minutes and by the end of it Jake was bright-eyed and alert, paws shifting impatiently, ready for anything. He seemed to know his troubles were over.

Roddy brought him back in ten days to have the stitches removed. It was, in fact, the very morning he was leaving the Darrowby district, and after I had picked the few loops of silk from the nicely healed wound I walked with him to the front door while Jake capered round our feet.

On the pavement outside Skeldale House the ancient pram stood in all its high, rusted dignity. Roddy pulled back the cover.

'Up, boy,' he murmured, and the big dog leaped effortlessly into his accustomed place.

Roddy took hold of the handle with both hands and as the autumn sunshine broke suddenly through the clouds it lit up a picture which had grown familiar and part of the daily scene. The golf jacket, the open shirt and brown chest, the handsome animal sitting up, looking around him with natural grace.

'Well, so long, Roddy,' I said. 'I suppose you'll be round these parts again.'

He turned and I saw that smile again. 'Aye, reckon ah'll be back.'

He gave a push and they were off, the strange vehicle creaking, Jake swaying gently as they went down the street. The memory came back to me of what I had seen under the cover that night in the surgery. The haversack, which would contain his razor, towel, soap and a few other things. The packet of tea and the thermos. And something else – a tiny dog collar. Could it have belonged to Jake as a pup or to another loved animal? It added a little more mystery to the man . . . and explained other things, too. That farmer had been right – all Roddy possessed was in that pram.

And it seemed it was all he desired, too, because as he turned the corner and disappeared from my view I could hear him whistling.

21

They had sent me to Eastchurch on the Isle of Sheppey and I knew it was the last stop.

As I looked along the disorderly line of men I realized I wouldn't be taking part in many more parades. And it came to me with a pang that at the Scarborough Initial Training Wing this would not have been classed as a parade at all. I could remember the ranks of blue outside the Grand Hotel, straight as the Grenadier Guards and every man standing stiffly, looking neither to left nor right. Our boots gleaming, buttons shining like gold and not a movement anywhere as the flight sergeant led the officer round on morning inspection.

I had moaned as loudly as anybody at the rigid discipline, the 'bull', the scrubbing and polishing, marching and drilling, but now that it had all gone it seemed good and meaningful and I missed it.

Here the files of airmen lounged, chatted among themselves and occasionally took a surreptitious drag at a cigarette as a sergeant out in front called the names from a list and gave us our leisurely instructions for the day.

This particular morning he was taking a long time over it, consulting sheaves of papers and making laboured notes with a pencil. A big Irishman on my right was becoming increasingly restive and finally he shouted testily:

'For — sake, sergeant, get us off this — square. Me — feet's killin' me!'

The sergeant didn't even look up. 'Shut your mouth, Brady,'

he replied. 'You'll get off the square when I say so and not before.'

It was like that at Eastchurch, the great filter tank of the RAF, where what I had heard described as the 'odds and sods' were finally sorted out. It was a big sprawling camp filled with a widely varied mixture of airmen who had one thing in common; they were all waiting – some of them for remuster, but most for discharge from the service.

There was a resigned air about the whole place, an acceptance of the fact that we were all just putting in time. There was a token discipline but it was of the most benign kind. And as I said, every man there was just waiting ... waiting ...

Little Ned Finch in his remote corner of the high Yorkshire Dales always seemed to me to be waiting, too. I could remember his boss yelling at him.

'For God's sake, shape up to t'job! You're not farmin' at all!' Mr Daggett grabbed hold of a leaping calf and glared in exasperation.

Ned gazed back at him impassively. His face registered no particular emotion, but in the pale blue eyes I read the expression that was always there – as though he was waiting for something to happen, but without much hope. He made a tentative attempt to catch a calf but was brushed aside, then he put his arms round the neck of another one, a chunky little animal of three months, and was borne along a few yards before being deposited on his back in the straw.

'Oh, dang it, do this one, Mr Herriot!' Mr Daggett barked, turning the hairy neck towards me. 'It looks as though I'll have to catch 'em all myself.'

I injected the animal. I was inoculating a batch of twenty with preventive pneumonia vaccine and Ned was suffering. With his diminutive stature and skinny, small-boned limbs he had always seemed to me to be in the wrong job; but he had been a farm worker all his life and he was over sixty now, grizzled, balding and slightly bent, but still battling on.

Mr Daggett reached out and as one of the shaggy creatures sped past he scooped the head into one of his great hands and seized the ear with the other. The little animal seemed to realize it was useless to struggle and stood unresisting as I inserted the needle. At the other end Ned put his knee against the calf's rear and listlessly pushed it against the wall. He wasn't doing much good and his boss gave him a withering glance.

We finished the bunch with hardly any help from the little man, and as we left the pen and came out into the yard Mr Daggett wiped his brow. It was a raw November day but he was sweating profusely and for a moment he leaned his gaunt six-foot frame against the wall as the wind from the bare moorland blew over him.

'By gaw, he's a useless little beggar is that,' he grunted. 'Ah don't know how ah put up with 'im.' He muttered to himself for a few moments, then gave tongue again. 'Hey, Ned!'

The little man who had been trailing aimlessly over the cobbles turned his pinched face and looked at him with his submissive but strangely expectant eyes.

'Get them bags o' corn up into the granary!' his boss ordered.

Wordlessly Ned went over to a cart and with an effort shouldered a sack of corn. As he painfully mounted the stone steps to the granary his frail little legs trembled and bent under the weight.

Mr Daggett shook his head and turned to me. His long cadaverous face was set in its usual cast of melancholy.

'You know what's wrong wi' Ned? he murmured confidentially.

'What do you mean?'

'Well, you know why 'e can't catch them calves?'

My own view was that Ned wasn't big enough or strong enough and anyway he was naturally ineffectual, but I shook my head.

'No,' I said. 'Why is it?'

'Well, I'll tell ye.' Mr Daggett glanced furtively across the yard then spoke from behind his hand. 'He's ower fond of t'bright lights.'

'Eh?'

'Ah'm tellin' ye, he's crazed over t'bright lights.'

'Bright ... what ... where ... ?'

Mr Daggett leaned closer. 'He gets over to Briston every night.'

'Briston ... ?' I looked across from the isolated farm to the village three miles away on the other side of the Dale. It was the only settlement in that bleak vista – a straggle of ancient houses dark and silent against the green fellside. I could recall that at night the oil lamps made yellow flickers of light in the windows but they weren't very bright. 'I don't understand.'

'Well . . . 'e gets into t'pub.'

'Ah, the pub.'

Mr Daggett nodded slowly and portentously but I was still puzzled. The Hulton Arms was a square kitchen where you could get a glass of beer and where a few old men played dominoes of an evening. It wasn't my idea of a den of vice.

'Does he get drunk there?' I asked.

'Nay, nay.' The farmer shook his head. 'It's not that. It's the hours 'e keeps.'

'Comes back late, eh?'

'Aye, that 'e does!' The eyes widened in their cavernous sockets. 'Sometimes 'e doesn't get back till 'alf past nine or ten o'clock!'

'Gosh, is that so?'

'Sure as ah'm standin' here. And there's another thing. He can't get out of 'is bed next day. Ah've done half a day's work before 'e starts.' He paused and glanced again across the yard. 'You can believe me or believe me not, but sometimes 'e isn't on the job till seven o'clock in t'morning!'

'Good heavens!'

He shrugged wearily. 'Aye well, you see how it is. Come into t'house, you'll want to wash your hands.'

In the huge flagged kitchen I bent low over the brown earthenware sink. Scar Farm was four hundred years old and the various tenants hadn't altered it much since the days of Henry the Eighth. Gnarled beams, rough whitewashed walls and hard wooden chairs. But comfort had never been important to Mr Daggett or his wife who was ladling hot water from the primitive boiler by the side of the fire and pouring it into her scrubbing bucket.

She clopped around over the flags in her clogs, hair pulled back tightly from her weathered face into a bun, a coarse sacking apron tied round her waist. She had no children but her life was one of constant activity; indoors or outside, she worked all the time.

At one end of the room wooden steps led up through a hole in the ceiling to a loft where Ned slept. That had been the little man's room for nearly fifty years, ever since he had come to work for Mr Daggett's father as a boy from school. And in all that time he had never travelled further than Darrowby, never done anything outside his daily routine. Wifeless, friendless, he plodded through his life, endlessly milking, feeding and mucking out, and waiting, I suspected with diminishing hope for something to happen.

With my hand on the car door I looked back at Scar Farm, at the sagging roof tiles, the great stone lintel over the door. It typified the harshness of the lives of the people within. Little Ned was no bargain as a stockman, and his boss's exasperation was understandable. Mr Daggett was not a cruel or an unjust man. He and his wife had been hardened and squeezed dry by the pitiless austerity of their existence in this lonely corner of the high Pennines.

There was no softness up here, no frills. The stone walls, sparse grass and stunted trees; the narrow road with its smears of cow muck. Everything was down to fundamentals, and it was a miracle to me that most of the Dalesmen were not like the Daggetts but cheerful and humorous.

But as I drove away, the sombre beauty of the place overwhelmed me. The lowering hillsides burst magically into life as a shaft of sunshine stabbed through the clouds, flooding the bare flanks with warm gold. Suddenly I was aware of the delicate shadings of green, the rich glowing bronze of the dead bracken spilling from the high tops, the whole peaceful majesty of my work-a-day world.

I hadn't far to drive to my next call – just about a mile – and it was in a vastly different atmosphere. Miss Tremayne, a rich lady from the south, had bought a tumbledown manor house and spent many thousands of pounds in converting it into a luxury home. As my feet crunched on the gravel I looked up at the large windows with their leaded panes, at the smooth, freshly-pointed stones.

Elsie opened the door to me. She was Miss Tremayne's cook-housekeeper, and one of my favourite people. Aged about fifty, no more than five feet high and as round as a ball with short bandy legs sticking out from beneath a tight black dress.

'Good morning, Elsie,' I said, and she burst into a peal of

laughter. This, more than her remarkable physical appearance, was what delighted me. She laughed uproariously at every statement and occurrence; in fact she laughed at the things she said herself.

'Come in, Mr Herriot, ha-ha-ha,' she said. 'It's been a bit nippy today, he-he, but I think it'll get out this afternoon, ho-ho-ho.'

All the mirth may have seemed somewhat unnecessary, and indeed, it made her rather difficult to understand, but the general effect was cheering. She led me into the drawing room and her mistress rose with some difficulty from her chair.

Miss Tremayne was elderly and half crippled with arthritis but bore her affliction without fuss.

'Ah, Mr Herriot,' she said. 'How good of you to come.' She put her head on one side and beamed at me as though I was the most delightful thing she had seen for a long time.

She, too, had a bubbling, happy personality, and since she owned three dogs, two cats and an elderly donkey I had come to know her very well in her six months' residence in the Dale.

My visit was to dress the donkey's overgrown hoofs, and a pair of clippers and a blacksmith's knife dangled from my right hand.

'Oh, put those grisly instruments down over there,' she said. 'Elsie's bringing some tea – I'm sure you've time for a cup.'

I sank willingly into ône of the brightly covered armchairs and was looking round the comfortable room when Elsie reappeared, gliding over the carpet as though on wheels. She put the tray on the table by my side.

'There's yer tea,' she said, and went into a paroxysm so hearty that she had to lean on the back of my chair. She had no visible neck and the laughter caused the fat little body to shake all over.

When she had recovered she rolled back into the kitchen and I heard her clattering about with pans. Despite her idiosyncrasies she was a wonderful cook and very efficient in all she did.

I spent a pleasant ten minutes with Miss Tremayne and the tea, then I went outside and attended to the donkey. When I had finished I made my way round the back of the house and as I was passing the kitchen I saw Elsie at the open window.

'Many thanks for the tea, Elsie,' I said.

The little woman gripped the sides of the sink to steady herself. 'Ha-ha-ha, that's all right. That's, he-he, quite all right, ha-ha-ho-ho-ho.'

Wonderingly I got into the car and as I drove away, the disturbing thought came to me that one day I might say something really witty to Elsie and cause her to do herself an injury.

I was called back to Mr Daggett's quite soon afterwards to see a cow which wouldn't get up. The farmer thought she was paralysed.

I drove there in a thin drizzle and the light was fading at about four o'clock in the afternoon when I arrived at Scar Farm.

When I examined the cow I was convinced she had just got herself into an awkward position in the stall with her legs jammed under the broken timbers of the partition.

'I think she's sulking, Mr Daggett,' I said. 'She's had a few goes at rising and now she's decided not to try any more. Some cows are like that.'

'Maybe you're right,' the farmer replied. 'She's allus been a stupid bitch.'

'And she's a big one, too. She'll take a bit of moving.' I lifted a rope from the byre wall and tied it round the hocks. 'I'll push the feet from the other side while you and Ned pull the legs round.'

'Pull ?' Mr Daggett gave the little man a sour look. 'He couldn't pull the skin off a rice puddin'.'

Ned said nothing, just gazed dully to his front, arms hanging limp. He looked as though he didn't care, wasn't even there with us. His mind was certainly elsewhere if his thoughts were mirrored in his eyes – vacant, unheeding, but as always, expectant.

I went behind the partition and thrust steadily at the feet while the men pulled. At least Mr Daggett pulled, mouth open, gasping with effort, while Ned leaned languidly on the rope.

Inch by inch the big animal came round till she was lying almost in the middle of the stall, but as I was about to call a halt the rope broke and Mr Daggett flew backwards on to the hard cobbles. Ned of course did not fall down because he hadn't been trying, and his employer, stretched flat, glared up at him with frustrated rage.

'Ye little bugger, ye let me do that all by meself! Ah don't know why ah bother with you, you're bloody useless.'

At that moment the cow, as I had expected, rose to her feet, and the farmer gesticulated at the little man. 'Well, go on, dang ye, get some straw and rub her legs! They'll be numb.'

Meekly Ned twisted some straw into a wisp and began to do a bit of massage. Mr Daggett got up stiffly, felt gingerly along his back, then walked up beside the cow to make sure the chain hadn't tightened round her neck. He was on his way back when the big animal swung round suddenly and brought her cloven hoof down solidly on the farmer's toe.

If he had been wearing heavy boots it wouldn't have been so bad, but his feet were encased in ancient cracked wellingtons which offered no protection.

'Ow! Ow! Ow!' yelled Mr Daggett, beating on the hairy back with his fists. 'Gerroff, ye awd bitch!' He heaved, pushed and writhed but the ten hundredweight of beef ground down inexorably.

The farmer was only released when the cow slid off his foot, and I know from experience that that sliding is the worst part.

Mr Daggett hopped around on one leg, nursing the bruised extremity in his hands. 'Bloody 'ell,' he moaned. 'Oh, bloody 'ell.'

Just then I happened to glance towards Ned and was amazed to see the apathetic little face crinkle suddenly into a wide grin of unholy glee. I couldn't recall him even smiling before, and my astonishment must have shown in my face because his boss whipped round suddenly and stared at him. As if by magic the sad mask slipped back into place and he went on with his rubbing.

Mr Daggett hobbled out to the car with me and as I was about to leave he nudged me.

'Look at 'im,' he whispered.

Ned, milk pail in hand, was bustling along the byre with unwonted energy.

His employer gave a bitter smile. 'It's t'only time 'e ever hurries. Can't wait to get out to t'pub.'

'Oh well, you say he doesn't get drunk. There can't be any harm in it.'

The deep sunk eyes held me. 'Don't you believe it. He'll come to a bad end gaddin' about the way 'e does.'

'But surely the odd glass of beer . . .'

'Ah but there's more than that to it.' He glanced around him. 'There's women!'

I laughed incredulously. 'Oh come now, Mr Daggett, what women ?'

'Over at t'pub,' he muttered. 'Them Bradley lasses.'

'The landlord's daughters ? Oh really, I can't believe . . .'

'All right, ye can say what ye like. He's got 'is eye on 'em. Ah knaw – ah've only been in that pub once but ah've seen for meself.'

I didn't know what to say, but in any case I had no opportunity because he turned and strode into the house.

Alone in the cold darkness I looked at the gaunt silhouette of the old farmhouse above me. In the dying light of the November day the rain streamed down the rough stones and the wind caught at the thin tendril of smoke from the chimney, hurling it in ragged streamers across the slate blue pallor of the western sky. The fell hung over everything, a black featureless bulk, oppressive and menacing.

Through the kitchen window I could see the oil lamp casting its dim light over the bare table, the cheerless hearth with its tiny flicker of fire. In the shadows at the far end the steps rose into Ned's loft and I could imagine the little figure clambering up to get changed and escape to Briston.

Across the valley the single street of the village was a broken grey thread in the gloom but in the cottage windows the lamps winked faintly. These were Ned Finch's bright lights and I could understand how he felt. After Scar Farm, Briston would be like Monte Carlo.

The image stayed in my mind so vividly that after two more calls that evening I decided to go a few miles out of my way as I returned homeward. I cut across the Dale and it was about half past eight when I drove into Briston. It was difficult to find the Hulton Arms because there was no lighted entrance, no attempt to advertise its presence, but I persevered because I had to find out what was behind Mr Daggett's tale of debauchery.

I located it at last. Just like the door of an ordinary house with a faded wooden sign hanging above it. Inside, the usual domino game was in progress, a few farmers sat chatting quietly. The Misses Bradley, plain but pleasant-faced women in their forties, sat on either side of the fire, and sure enough there was Ned with a half pint glass in front of him.

I sat down by his side. 'Hello, Ned.'

'Now then, Mr Herriot,' he murmured absently, glancing at me with his strange expectant eyes.

One of the Bradley ladies put down her knitting and came over. 'Pint of bitter, please,' I said. 'What will you have, Ned ?'

'Nay, thank ye, Mr Herriot. This'll do for me. It's me second and ah'm not a big drinker, tha knows.'

Miss Bradley laughed. 'Yes, he nobbut has 'is two glasses a night, but he enjoys them, don't you, Ned ?'

'That's right, ah do.' He looked up at her and she smiled kindly down at him before going for my beer.

He took a sip at his glass. 'Ah really come for t'company, Mr Herriot.'

'Yes, of course,' I said. I knew what he meant. He probably sat on his own most of the time, but around him was warmth and comfort and friendliness. A great log sent flames crackling up to the wide chimney, there was electric light and shining mirrors with whisky slogans painted on their surface. It wasn't anything like Scar Farm.

The little man said very little. He spun out his drink for another hour, looking around him as the dominoes clicked and I lowered another contemplative pint. The Misses Bradley knitted and brewed tea in a big black kettle over the fire and when they had to get up to serve their customers they occasionally patted Ned playfully on the cheek as they passed.

By the time he tipped down the last drop and rose to go it was a quarter to ten and he still had to cycle across to the other side of the Dale. Another late night for Ned.

It was a Tuesday lunchtime in early spring. Helen always cooked steak and kidney pie on Tuesdays and I used to think about it all morning on my rounds. My thoughts that morning had been particularly evocative because lambing had started and I had spent most of the time in my shirt sleeves in the biting wind as my hunger grew and grew.

Helen cut into her blissful creation and began to scoop the fragrant contents on to my plate.

'I met Miss Tremayne in the market place this morning, Jim.'

'Oh yes ?' I was almost drooling as my wife stopped shovelling out the pie, sliced open some jacket potatoes and dropped pats of farm butter on to the steaming surfaces.

'Yes, she wants you to go out there this afternoon and put some canker drops in Wilberforce's ears if you have time.'

'Oh I have time for that,' I said. Wilberforce was Miss Tremayne's ancient tabby cat and it was just the kind of job I wanted after my arm-aching morning.

I was raising a luscious forkful when Helen spoke again. 'Oh, and she had an interesting item of news.'

'Really ?' But I had begun to chew and my thoughts were distant.

'Its' about the little woman who works for her – Elsie. You know her ?'

I nodded and took another mouthful. 'Of course, of course.'

'Well, it's quite unexpected, I suppose, but Elsie's getting married.'

I choked on my pie. 'What!'

'It's true. And maybe you know the bridegroom.'

'Tell me.'

'He works on one of the neighbouring farms. His name is Ned Finch.'

This time my breath was cut off completely and Helen had to beat me on the back as I spluttered and retched. It wasn't until an occluding morsel of potato skin had shot down my nose that I was able to utter a weak croak. 'Ned Finch ?'

'That's what she said.'

I finished my lunch in a dream, but by the end of it I had accepted the extraordinary fact. Helen and Miss Tremayne were two sensible people – there couldn't be any mistake. And yet . . . even as I drew up outside the old Manor House a feeling of unreality persisted.

Elsie opened the door as usual. I looked at her for a moment.

'What's this I hear, Elsie?'

She started a giggle which rapidly spread over her spherical frame.

I put my hand on her shoulder. 'Is it true?'

The giggle developed into a mighty gale of laughter, and if she hadn't been holding the handle I am sure she would have fallen over.

'Aye, it's right enough,' she gasped. 'Ah've found a man at last and ah'm goin' to get wed!' She leaned helplessly on the door.

'Well, I'm pleased to hear it, Elsie. I hope you'll be very happy.'

She hadn't the strength to speak but merely nodded as she lay against the door. Then she led me to the drawing room.

'In ye go,' she chuckled. 'Ah'll bring ye some tea.'

Miss Tremayne rose to greet me with parted lips and shining eyes. 'Oh, Mr Herriot, have you heard?'

'Yes, but how ...?'

'It all started when I asked Mr Daggett for some fresh eggs. He sent Ned on his bicycle with the eggs and it was like fate.'

'Well, how wonderful.'

'Yes, and I actually saw it happen. Ned walked in that door with his basket, Elsie was clearing the table here, and, Mr Herriot—' She clasped her hands under her chin, smiled ecstatically and her eyes rolled upwards. 'Oh, Mr Herriot, it was love at first sight!'

'Yes ... yes, indeed. Marvellous!'

'And ever since that day Ned has been calling round and now he comes every evening and sits with Elsie in the kitchen. Isn't it romantic!'

'It certainly is. And when did they decide to get married?'

'Oh, he popped the question within a month, and I'm so happy for Elsie because Ned is such a dear little man, don't you think so?'

'Yes, he is.' I said. 'He's a very nice chap.'

Elsie simpered and tittered her way in with the tea then put her hand over her face and fled in confusion, and as Miss Tremayne began to pour I sank into one of the armchairs and lifted Wilberforce on to my lap.

The big cat purred as I instilled a few drops of lotion into his ear. He had a chronic canker condition – not very bad but now and then it became painful and needed treatment. It was because Miss Tremayne didn't like putting the lotion in that I was pressed into service.

As I turned the ear over and gently massaged the oily liquid into the depths, Wilberforce groaned softly with pleasure and rubbed his cheek against my hand. He loved this anointing of the tender area beyond his reach and when I had finished he curled up on my knee.

I leaned back and sipped my tea. At that moment, with my back and shoulders weary and my hands red and chapped with countless washings on the open hillsides this seemed to be veterinary practice at its best.

Miss Tremayne continued. 'We shall have a little reception after the wedding and then the happy couple will take up residence here.'

'You mean, in this house?'

'Yes, of course. There's heaps of room in this big old place, and I have furnished two rooms for them on the east side. I'm sure they'll be very comfortable. Oh, I'm so excited about it all!'

She refilled my cup. 'Before you go you must let Elsie show you where they are going to live.'

On my way out the little woman took me through to the far end of the house.

'This, hee-hee-hee,' she said, 'is where we'll sit of a night, and this, ha-ha-ho-ho, oh dear me, is our bedroom.' She staggered around for a bit, wiped her eyes and turned to me for my opinion.

'It's really lovely, Elsie,' I said.

There were bright carpets, chairs with flowered covers and a fine mahogany-ended bed. It was nothing like the loft.

And as I looked at Elsie I realized the things Ned would see in his bride. Laughter, warmth, vivacity, and – I had no doubt at all – beauty and glamour.

I seemed to get round to most farms that lambing time and in due course I landed at Mr Daggett's. I delivered a fine pair of twins for him but it didn't seem to cheer him at all. Lifting the towel from the grass he handed it to me.

'Well, what did ah tell ye about Ned, eh? Got mixed up wi' a woman just like ah said.' He sniffed disapprovingly. 'All that rakin' and chasin' about – ah knew he'd get into mischief at t'finish.'

I walked back over the sunlit fields to the farm and as I passed the byre door Ned came out pushing a wheelbarrow.

'Good morning, Ned,' I said.

He glanced up at me in his vague way. 'How do, Mr Herriot.'

There was something different about him and it took me a few moments to discern what it was; his eyes had lost the expectant look which had been there for so long, and, after all, that was perfectly natural.

Because it had happened at last for Ned.

22

Despite the crowds of men milling around Eastchurch I felt cut off and apart. It made me think of old Mr Potts from my veterinary days. He must have felt like that.

'How are you, Mr Herriot?'

Ordinary words, but the eagerness, almost desperation in the old man's voice made them urgent and meaningful.

I saw him nearly every day. In my unpredictable life it was difficult to do anything regularly but I did like a stroll by the river before lunch and so did my beagle, Sam. That was when we met Mr Potts and Nip, his elderly sheepdog – they seemed to have the same habits as us. His house backed on to the riverside fields and he spent a lot of time just walking around with his dog.

Many retired farmers kept a bit of land and a few stock to occupy their minds and ease the transition from their arduous existence to day-long leisure, but Mr Potts had bought a little bungalow with a scrap of garden and it was obvious that time dragged.

Probably his health had dictated this. As he faced me he leaned on his stick and his bluish cheeks rose and fell with his breathing. He was a heart case if ever I saw one.

'I'm fine, Mr Potts,' I replied. 'And how are things with you ?'

'Nobbut middlin', lad. Ah soon get short o' wind.' He coughed a couple of times then asked the inevitable question.

'And what have you been doin' this mornin' ?' That was when his eyes grew intent and wide. He really wanted to know.

I thought for a moment. 'Well now, let's see.' I always tried to give him a detailed answer because I knew it meant a lot to him and brought back the life he missed so much. 'I've done a couple of cleansings, seen a lame bullock, treated two cows with mastitis and another with milk fever.'

He nodded eagerly at every word.

'By gaw!' he exclaimed. 'It's a beggar, that milk fever. When I were a lad, good cows used to die like flies with it. Allus good milkers after their third or fourth calf. Couldn't get to their feet and we used to dose 'em with all sorts, but they died, every one of 'em.'

'Yes,' I said. 'It must have been heartbreaking in those days.'

'But then—' He smiled delightedly, digging a forefinger into my chest. 'Then we started blowin' up their udders wi' a bicycle pump, and d'you know – they jumped up and walked away. Like magic it were.' His eyes sparkled at the memory.

'I know, Mr Potts, I've blown up a few myself, only I didn't use a bicycle pump – I had a special little inflation apparatus.'

That black box with its shining cylinders and filter is now in my personal museum, and it is the best place for it. It had got me out of some difficult situations but in the background there had always been the gnawing dread of transmitting tuberculosis. I had heard of it happening and was glad that calcium borogluconate had arrived.

As we spoke, Sam and Nip played on the grass beside us. I watched as the beagle frisked round the old animal while Nip pawed at him stiff-jointedly, his tail waving with pleasure. You could see that he enjoyed these meetings as much as his master and for a brief time the years fell away from him as he rolled on his back with Sam astride him, nibbling gently at his chest.

I walked with the old farmer as far as the little wooden bridge, then I had to turn for home. I watched the two of them pottering slowly over the narrow strip of timber to the other side of the river. Sam and I had our work pressing, but they had nothing else to do.

I used to see Mr Potts at other times, too. Wandering aimlessly among the stalls on market days or standing on the fringe of the group of farmers who always gathered in front of the Drovers' Arms to meet cattle dealers, cow feed merchants, or just to talk business among themselves.

Or I saw him at the auction mart, leaning on his stick, listening to the rapid-fire chanting of the auctioneer, watching listlessly as the beasts were bought and sold. And all the time I knew there was an emptiness in him, because there were none of his cattle in the stalls, none of his sheep in the long rows of pens. He was out of it all, old and done.

I saw him the day before he died. It was in the usual place and I was standing at the river's edge watching a heron rising from a rush-lined island and flapping lazily away over the fields.

The old man stopped as he came abreast of me and the two dogs began their friendly wrestling.

'Well now, Mr Herriot.' He paused and bowed his head over the stick which he had dug into the grass of his farm for half a century. 'What have you been doin' today ?'

Perhaps his cheeks were a deeper shade of blue and the breath whistled through his pursed lips as he exhaled, but I can't recall that he looked any worse than usual.

'I'll tell you, Mr Potts,' I said. 'I'm feeling a bit weary. I ran into a real snorter of a foaling this morning – took me over two hours and I ache all over.'

'Foaling, eh ? Foal would be laid wrong, I reckon ?'

'Yes, crossways on, and I had a struggle to turn it.'

'By gaw, yes, it's hard work is that.' He smiled reminiscently. 'Doesta remember that Clydesdale mare you foaled at ma place ? Must 'ave been one of your first jobs when you came to Darrowby.'

'Of course I do,' I replied. And I remembered too, how kind the old man had been. Seeing I was young and green and unsure of myself he had taken pains, in his quiet way, to put me at my ease and give me confidence. 'Yes,' I went on, 'it was late on a Sunday night and we had a right tussle with it. There was just the two of us but we managed, didn't we ?'

He squared his shoulders and for a moment his eyes looked past me at something I couldn't see. 'Aye, that's right. We made a job of 'er, you and me. Ah could push and pull a bit then.'

'You certainly could. There's no doubt about that.'

He sucked the air in with difficulty and blew it out again with that peculiar pursing of the lips. Then he turned to me with a strange dignity.

'They were good days, Mr Herriot, weren't they ?'

'They were, Mr Potts, they were indeed.'

'Aye, aye.' He nodded slowly. 'Ah've had a lot o' them days. Hard but good.' He looked down at his dog. 'And awd Nip shared 'em with me, didn't ye, lad ?'

His words took me back to the very first time I had seen Mr Potts. He was perched on a stool, milking one of his few cows, his cloth-capped head thrusting into the hairy flank, and as he pulled at the teats old Nip dropped a stone on the toe of his boot. The farmer reached down, lifted the stone between two fingers and flicked it out through the open door into the yard. Nip scurried delightedly after it and was back within seconds, dropping the stone on the boot and panting hopefully.

He wasn't disappointed. His master repeated the throw automatically as if it was something he did all the time, and as I watched it happening again and again I realized that this was a daily ritual between the two. I had a piercing impression of infinite patience and devotion.

'Right, then, Mr Herriot, we'll be off,' Mr Potts said, jerking me back to the present. 'Come on, Nip.' He waved his stick and I watched him till a low-hanging willow branch hid man and dog from my sight.

That was the last time I saw him. Next day the man at the petrol pumps mumbled casually. 'See old Mr Potts got his time in, eh ?'

And that was it. There was no excitement, and only a handful of his old friends turned up at the funeral.

For me it was a stab of sorrow. Another familiar face gone, and I should miss him as my busy life went on. I knew our daily conversations had cheered him but I felt with a sad finality that there was nothing else I could do for Mr Potts.

It was about a fortnight later and as I opened the gate to let Sam into the riverside fields I glanced at my watch. Twelve-thirty – plenty of time for our pre-lunch walk and the long stretch of green was empty. Then I noticed a single dog away on the left. It was Nip, and as I watched he got up, took a few indeterminate steps over the grass then turned and sat down again at the gate of his back garden.

Instead of taking my usual route I cut along behind the houses till I reached the old dog. He had been looking around him aimlessly but when we came up to him he seemed to come to life, sniffing Sam over and wagging his tail at me.

On the other side of the gate Mrs Potts was doing a bit of weeding, bending painfully as she plied her trowel.

'How are you, Mrs Potts?' I said.

With an effort she straightened up. 'Oh, not too bad, thank you, Mr Herriot.' She came over and leaned on the gate. 'I see you're lookin' at the awd dog. My word he's missin' his master.'

I didn't say anything and she went on. 'He's eating all right and I can give him plenty of good food, but what I can't do is take 'im for walks.' She rubbed her back. 'I'm plagued with rheumaticks, Mr Herriot, and it takes me all my time to get around the house and garden.'

'I can understand that,' I said. 'And I don't suppose he'll walk by himself.'

'Nay, he won't. There's the path he went along every day.' She pointed to the winding strip of beaten earth among the grass. 'But he won't go more'n a few yards.'

'Ah well, dogs like a bit of company just the same as we do.' I bent and ran my hand over the old animal's head and ears. 'How would you like to come with us, Nip?'

I set off along the path and he followed unhesitatingly, trotting alongside Sam with swinging tail.

'Eee, look!' the old lady cried. 'Isn't that grand to see!'

I followed his usual route down to the river where the water ran dark and silent under the branches of the gnarled willows. Then we went over the bridge and in front of us the river widened into pebbly shallows and murmured and chattered among the stones.

It was peaceful down there with only the endless water sound and the piping of birds in my ears and the long curtain of leaves parting here and there to give glimpses of the green flanks of the fells.

I watched the two dogs frisking ahead of me and the decision came to me quite naturally; I would do this regularly. From that day I altered my route and went along behind the houses first. Nip was happy again, Sam loved the whole idea, and for me there was a strange comfort in the knowledge that there was still something I could do for Mr Potts.

23

I had plenty of time on my hands at Eastchurch, plenty of time to think, and like most servicemen I thought of home. Only my home wasn't there any more.

When I left Darrowby Helen had gone back to live with her father and the little rooms under the tiles of Skeldale House would be empty and dusty now. But they lived on in my mind, clear in every detail.

I could see the ivy-fringed window looking over the tumble of roofs to the green hills, our few pieces of furniture, the bed and side table and the old wardrobe which only stayed shut with the aid of one of my socks jammed in the door. Strangely, it was that dangling woollen toe which gave me the sharpest stab as I remembered.

And even though it was all gone I could hear the bedside radio playing, my wife's voice from the other side of the fire and on that winter evening Tristan shouting up the stairs from the passage far below.

'Jim! Jim!'

I went out and stuck my head over the banisters. 'What is it, Triss?'

'Sorry to bother you, Jim, but could you come down for a minute?' The upturned face had an anxious look.

I went down the long flights of steps two at a time and when I arrived slightly breathless on the ground floor Tristan beckoned me through to the consulting room at the back of the house. A teenage girl was standing by the table, her hand resting on a stained roll of blanket.

'It's a cat,' Tristan said. He pulled back a fold of the blanket and I looked down at a large, deeply striped tabby. At least he would have been large if he had had any flesh on his bones, but ribs and pelvis stood out painfully through the fur and as I passed my hand over the motionless body I could feel only a thin covering of skin.

Tristan cleared his throat. 'There's something else, Jim.'

I looked at him curiously. For once he didn't seem to have a joke in him. I watched as he gently lifted one of the cat's hind legs and rolled the abdomen into view. There was a gash on the ventral surface through which a coiled cluster of intestines spilled grotesquely on to the cloth. I was still shocked and staring when the girl spoke.

'I saw this cat sittin' in the dark, down Brown's yard. I thought 'e looked skinny, like, and a bit quiet and I bent down to give 'im a pat. Then I saw 'e was badly hurt and I went home for a blanket and brought 'im round to you.'

'That was kind of you,' I said. 'Have you any idea who he belongs to?'

The girl shook her head. 'No, he looks like a stray to me.'

'He does indeed.' I dragged my eyes away from the terrible wound. 'You're Marjorie Simpson, aren't you?'

'Yes.'

'I know your Dad well. He's our postman.'

'That's right.' She gave a half-smile, then her lips trembled. 'Well, I reckon I'd better leave 'im with you. You'll be goin' to put him out of his misery. There's nothing anybody can do about . . . about that?'

I shrugged and shook my head. The girl's eyes filled with tears, she stretched out a hand and touched the emaciated animal then turned and walked quickly to the door.

'Thanks again, Marjorie,' I called after the retreating back. 'And don't worry – we'll look after him.'

In the silence that followed, Tristan and I looked down at the shattered animal. Under the surgery lamp it was all too easy to see. He had almost been disembowelled and the pile of intestines was covered in dirt and mud.

'What d'you think did this?' Tristan said at length. 'Has he been run over?'

'Maybe,' I replied. 'Could be anything. An attack by a big dog or somebody could have kicked him or struck him.' All things were possible with cats because some people seemed to regard them as fair game for any cruelty.

Tristan nodded. 'Anyway, whatever happened, he must have been on the verge of starvation. He's a skeleton. I bet he's wandered miles from home.'

'Ah well,' I signed. 'There's only one thing to do. Those guts are perforated in several places. It's hopeless.'

Tristan didn't say anything but he whistled under his breath and drew the tip of his forefinger again and again across the furry cheek. And, unbelievably, from somewhere in the scraggy chest a gentle purring arose.

The young man looked at me, round eyes. 'My God, do you hear that?'

'Yes . . . amazing in that condition. He's a good-natured cat.'

Tristan, head bowed, continued his stroking. I knew how he felt because, although he preserved a cheerfully hard-boiled attitude to our patients he couldn't kid me about one thing; he had a soft spot for cats. Even now, when we are both around the sixty mark, he often talks to me over a beer about the cat he has had for many years. It is a typical relationship – they tease each other unmercifully – but it is based on real affection.

'It's no good, Triss,' I said gently. 'It's got to be done.' I reached for the syringe but something in me rebelled against plunging a needle into that mutilated body. Instead I pulled a fold of the blanket over the cat's head.

'Pour a little ether on to the cloth,' I said. 'He'll just sleep away.'

Wordlessly Tristan unscrewed the cap of the ether bottle and poised it above the head. Then from under the shapeless heap of blanket we heard it again; the deep purring which increased in volume till it boomed in our ears like a distant motor cycle.

Tristan was like a man turned to stone, hand gripping the

bottle rigidly, eyes staring down at the mound of cloth from which the purring rose in waves of warm friendly sound.

At last he looked up at me and gulped. 'I don't fancy this much, Jim. Can't we do something?'

'You mean, put that lot back?'

'Yes.'

'But the bowels are damaged – they're like a sieve in parts.'

'We could stitch them, couldn't we?'

I lifted the blanket and looked again. 'Honestly, Triss, I wouldn't know where to start. And the whole thing is filthy.'

He didn't say anything, but continued to look at me steadily.

And I didn't need much persuading. I had no more desire to pour ether on to that comradely purring than he had.

'Come on, then,' I said. 'We'll have a go.'

With the oxygen bubbling and the cat's head in the anaesthetic mask we washed the whole prolapse with warm saline. We did it again and again but it was impossible to remove every fragment of caked dirt. Then we started the painfully slow business of stitching the many holes in the tiny intestines, and here I was glad of Tristan's nimble fingers which seemed better able to manipulate the small round-bodied needles than mine.

Two hours and yards of catgut later, we dusted the patched up peritoneal surface with sulphonamide and pushed the entire mass back into the abdomen. When I had sutured muscle layers and skin everything looked tidy but I had a nasty feeling of sweeping undesirable things under the carpet. The extensive damage, all that contamination – peritonitis was inevitable.

'He's alive, anyway, Triss,' I said as we began to wash the instruments. 'We'll put him on to sulphapyridine and keep our fingers crossed.' There were still no antibiotics at that time but the new drug was a big advance.

The door opened and Helen came in. 'You've been a long time, Jim.' She walked over to the table and looked down at the sleeping cat. 'What a poor skinny little thing. He's all bones.'

'You should have seen him when he came in.' Tristan switched off the sterilizer and screwed shut the valve on the anaesthetic machine. 'He looks a lot better now.'

She stroked the little animal for a moment. 'Is he badly injured?'

'I'm afraid so, Helen,' I said. 'We've done our best for him but I honestly don't think he has much chance.'

'What a shame. And he's pretty, too. Four white feet and all those unusual colours.' With her finger she traced the faint bands of auburn and copper-gold among the grey and black.

Tristan laughed. 'Yes, I think that chap has a ginger tom somewhere in his ancestry.'

Helen smiled, too, but absently, and I noticed a broody look about her. She hurried out to the stock room and returned with an empty box.

'Yes . . . yes . . .' she said thoughtfully. 'I can make a bed in this box for him and he'll sleep in our room, Jim.'

'He will?'

'Yes, he must be warm, mustn't he?'

'Of course.'

Later, in the darkness of our bedsitter, I looked from my pillow at a cosy scene; Sam in his basket on one side of the flickering fire and the cat cushioned and blanketed in his box on the other.

As I floated off into sleep it was good to know that my patient was so comfortable, but I wondered if he would be alive in the morning . . .

I knew he was alive at 7.30 a.m. because my wife was already up and talking to him. I trailed across the room in my pyjamas and the cat and I looked at each other. I rubbed him under the chin and he opened his mouth in a rusty miaow. But he didn't try to move.

'Helen,' I said. 'This little thing is tied together inside with catgut. He'll have to live on fluids for a week and even then he probably won't make it. If he stays up here you'll be spooning milk into him umpteen times a day.'

'Okay, okay.' She had that broody look again.

It wasn't only milk she spooned into him over the next few days. Beef essence, strained broth and a succession of sophisticated baby foods found their way down his throat at regular intervals. One lunch time I found Helen kneeling by the box.

'We shall call him Oscar,' she said.

'You mean we're keeping him?'

'Yes.'

I am fond of cats but we already had a dog in our cramped

212

quarters and I could see difficulties. Still I decided to let it go.

'Why Oscar?'

'I don't know.' Helen tipped a few drops of chop gravy on to the little red tongue and watched intently as he swallowed.

One of the things I like about women is their mystery, the unfathomable part of them, and I didn't press the matter further. But I was pleased at the way things were going. I had been giving the sulphapyridine every six hours and taking the temperature night and morning, expecting all the time to encounter the roaring fever, the vomiting and the tense abdomen of peritonitis. But it never happened.

It was as though Oscar's animal instinct told him he had to move as little as possible because he lay absolutely still day after day and looked up at us – and purred.

His purr became part of our lives and when he eventually left his bed, sauntered through to our kitchen and began to sample Sam's dinner of meat and biscuit it was a moment of triumph. And I didn't spoil it by wondering if he was ready for solid food; I felt he knew.

From then on it was a sheer joy to watch the furry scarecrow fill out and grow strong, and as he ate and ate and the flesh spread over his bones the true beauty of his coat showed in the glossy medley of auburn, black and gold. We had a handsome cat on our hands.

Once Oscar had recovered, Tristan was a regular visitor.

He probably felt, and rightly, that he, more than I, had saved Oscar's life in the first place and he used to play with him for long periods. His favourite ploy was to push his leg round the corner of the table and withdraw it repeatedly just as the cat pawed at it.

Oscar was justifiably irritated by this teasing but showed his character by lying in wait for Tristan one night and biting him smartly in the ankle before he could start his tricks.

From my own point of view Oscar added many things to our ménage. Sam was delighted with him and the two soon became firm friends, Helen adored him and each evening I thought afresh that a nice cat washing his face by the hearth gave extra comfort to a room.

Oscar had been established as one of the family for several

weeks when I came in from a late call to find Helen waiting for me with a stricken face.

'What's happened?' I asked.

'It's Oscar – he's gone!'

'Gone? what do you mean?'

'Oh, Jim, I think he's run away.'

I stared at her. 'He wouldn't do that. He often goes down to the garden at night. Are you sure he isn't there?'

'Absolutely. I've searched right into the yard. I've even had a walk round the town. And remember.' Her chin quivered. 'He ... he ran away from somewhere before.'

I looked at my watch. 'Ten o'clock. Yes, that is strange. He shouldn't be out at this time.'

As I spoke the front door bell jangled. I galloped down the stairs and as I rounded the corner in the passage I could see Mrs Heslington, the vicar's wife, through the glass. I threw open the door. She was holding Oscar in her arms.

'I believe this is your cat, Mr Herriot,' she said.

'It is indeed, Mrs Heslington. Where did you find him?'

She smiled. 'Well, it was rather odd. We were having a meeting of the Mothers' Union at the church house and we noticed the cat sitting there in the room.'

'Just sitting...?'

'Yes, as though he were listening to what we were saying and enjoying it all. It was unusual. When the meeting ended I thought I'd better bring him along to you.'

'I'm most grateful, Mrs Heslington.' I snatched Oscar and tucked him under my arm. 'My wife is distraught – she thought he was lost.'

It was a little mystery. Why should he suddenly take off like that? But since he showed no change in his manner over the ensuing week we put it out of our minds.

Then one evening a man brought in a dog for a distemper inoculation and left the front door open. When I went up to our flat I found that Oscar had disappeared again. This time Helen and I scoured the market place and side alleys in vain and when we returned at half past nine we were both despondent. It was nearly eleven and we were thinking of bed when the door bell rang.

It was Oscar again, this time resting on the ample stomach of Jack Newbould. Jack was leaning against a doorpost and the fresh country air drifting in from the dark street was richly intermingled with beer fumes.

Jack was a gardener at one of the big houses. He hiccuped gently and gave me a huge benevolent smile. 'Brought your cat, Mr Herriot.'

'Gosh, thanks, Jack!' I said, scooping up Oscar gratefully. 'Where the devil did you find him?'

'Well, s'matter o' fact, 'e sort of found me.'

'What do you mean?'

Jack closed his eyes for a few moments before articulating carefully. 'Thish is a big night, tha knows, Mr Herriot. Darts championship. Lots of t'lads round at t'Dog and Gun – lotsh and lotsh of 'em. Big gatherin'.'

'And our cat was there?'

'Aye, he were there, all right. Sittin' among t'lads. Shpent t'whole evenin' with us.'

'Just sat there, eh?'

'That 'e did.' Jack giggled reminiscently. 'By gaw 'e enjoyed isself. Ah gave 'im a drop o' best bitter out of me own glass and once or twice ah thought 'e was goin' to have a go at chuckin' a dart. He's some cat.' He laughed again.

As I bore Oscar upstairs I was deep in thought. What was going on here? These sudden desertions were upsetting Helen and I felt they could get on my nerves in time.

I didn't have long to wait till the next one. Three nights later he was missing again. This time Helen and I didn't bother to search – we just waited.

He was back earlier than usual. I heard the door bell at nine o'clock. It was the elderly Miss Simpson peering through the glass. And she wasn't holding Oscar – he was prowling on the mat waiting to come in.

Miss Simpson watched with interest as the cat stalked inside and made for the stairs. 'Ah, good, I'm so glad he's come home safely. I knew he was your cat and I've been intrigued by his behaviour all evening.'

'Where . . . may I ask?'

'Oh, at the Women's Institute. He came in shortly after we started and stayed till the end.'

'Really ? What exactly was your programme, Miss Simpson ?'

'Well, there was a bit of committee stuff, then a short talk with lantern slides by Mr Walters from the water company and we finished with a cake-making competition.'

'Yes . . . yes . . . and what did Oscar do ?'

She laughed. 'Mixed with the company, apparently enjoyed the slides and showed great interest in the cakes.'

'I see. And you didn't bring him home ?'

'No, he made his own way here. As you know, I have to pass your house and I merely rang your bell to make sure you knew he had arrived.'

'I'm obliged to you, Miss Simpson. We were a little worried.'

I mounted the stairs in record time. Helen was sitting with the cat on her knee and she looked up as I burst in.

'I know about Oscar now,' I said.

'Know what ?'

'Why he goes on these nightly outings. He's not running away – he's visiting.'

'Visiting ?'

'Yes,' I said. 'Don't you see ? He likes getting around, he loves people, especially in groups, and he's interested in what they do. He's a natural mixer.'

Helen looked down at the attractive mound of fur curled on her lap. 'Of course . . . that's it . . . he's a socialite!'

'Exactly, a high stepper!'

'A cat-about-town!'

It all afforded us some innocent laughter and Oscar sat up and looked at us with evident pleasure, adding his own throbbing purr to the merriment. But for Helen and me there was a lot of relief behind it; ever since our cat had started his excursions there had been the gnawing fear that we would lose him, and now we felt secure.

From that night our delight in him increased. There was endless joy in watching this facet of his character unfolding. He did the social round meticulously, taking in most of the activities of the town. He became a familiar figure at whist drives, jumble sales, school concerts and scout bazaars. Most of the time he was made welcome, but was twice ejected from meetings of the Rural

District Council who did not seem to relish the idea of a cat sitting in on their deliberations.

At first I was apprehensive about his making his way through the streets but I watched him once or twice and saw that he looked both ways before tripping daintily across. Clearly he had excellent traffic sense and this made me feel that his original injury had not been caused by a car.

Taking it all in all, Helen and I felt that it was a kind stroke of fortune which had brought Oscar to us. He was a warm and cherished part of our home life. He added to our happiness.

When the blow fell it was totally unexpected.

I was finishing the evening surgery. I looked round the door and saw only a man and two little boys.

'Next please,' I said.

The man stood up. He had no animal with him. He was middle-aged, with the rough weathered face of a farm worker. He twirled a cloth cap nervously in his hands.

'Mr Herriot ?' he said.

'Yes, what can I do for you ?'

He swallowed and looked me straight in the eyes. 'Ah think you've got ma cat.'

'What ?'

'Ah lost ma cat a bit since.' He cleared his throat. 'We used to live at Missdon but ah got a job as ploughman to Mr Horne of Wederly. It was after we moved to Wederly that t'cat went missin.' Ah reckon he was tryin' to find 'is way back to his old home.'

'Wederly ? That's on the other side of Brawton – over thirty miles away.'

'Aye, ah knaw, but cats is funny things.'

'But what makes you think I've got him ?'

He twisted the cap around a bit more. 'There's a cousin o' mine lives in Darrowby and ah heard tell from 'im about this cat that goes around to meetin's. I 'ad to come. We've been huntin' everywhere.'

'Tell me,' I said. 'This cat you lost. What did he look like ?'

'Grey and black and sort o' gingery. Right bonny 'e was. And 'e was allus goin' out to gatherin's.'

A cold hand clutched at my heart. 'You'd better come upstairs. Bring the boys with you.'

Helen was putting some coal on the fire of the bedsitter.

'Helen,' I said. 'This is Mr – er – I'm sorry, I don't know your name.'

'Gibbons, Sep Gibbons. They called me Septimus because ah was the seventh in family and it looks like ah'm goin' t'same way 'cause we've got six already. These are our two youngest.' The two boys, obvious twins of about eight, looked up at us solemnly.

I wished my heart would stop hammering. 'Mr Gibbons thinks Oscar is his. He lost his cat some time ago.'

My wife put down her little shovel. 'Oh . . . oh . . . I see.' She stood very still for a moment then smiled faintly. 'Do sit down. Oscar's in the kitchen, I'll bring him through.'

She went out and reappeared with the cat in her arms. She hadn't got through the door before the little boys gave tongue.

'Tiger!' they cried. 'Oh, Tiger, Tiger!'

The man's face seemed lit from within. He walked quickly across the floor and ran his big work-roughened hand along the fur.

'Hullo, awd lad,' he said, and turned to me with a radiant smile. 'It's 'im, Mr Herriot, It's 'im awright, and don't 'e look well!'

'You call him Tiger, eh?' I said.

'Aye,' he replied happily. 'It's them gingery stripes. The kids called 'im that. They were broken-hearted when we lost 'im.'

As the two little boys rolled on the floor our Oscar rolled with them, pawing playfully, purring with delight.

Sep Gibbons sat down again. 'That's the way 'e allus went on wi' the family. They used to play with 'im for hours. By gaw we did miss 'im. He were a right favourite.'

I looked at the broken nails on the edge of the cap, at the decent, honest, uncomplicated Yorkshire face so like the many I had grown to like and respect. Farm men like him got thirty shillings a week in those days and it was reflected in the threadbare jacket, the cracked, shiny boots and the obvious hand-me-downs of the boys.

But all three were scrubbed and tidy, the man's face like a red beacon, the children's knees gleaming and their hair carefully

218

slicked across their foreheads. They looked like nice people to me. I didn't know what to say.

Helen said it for me. 'Well, Mr Gibbons.' Her tone had an unnatural brightness. 'You'd better take him.'

The man hesitated. 'Now then, are ye sure, Missis Herriot?'

'Yes . . . yes, I'm sure. He was your cat first.'

'Aye, but some folks 'ud say finders keepers or summat like that. Ah didn't come 'ere to demand 'im back or owt of t'sort.'

'I know you didn't, Mr Gibbons, but you've had him all those years and you've searched for him so hard. We couldn't possibly keep him from you.'

He nodded quickly. 'Well, that's right good of ye.' He paused for a moment, his face serious, then he stooped and picked Oscar up. 'We'll have to be off if we're goin' to catch the eight o'clock bus.'

Helen reached forward, cupped the cat's head in her hands and looked at him steadily for a few seconds. Then she patted the boys' heads. 'You'll take good care of him, won't you?'

'Aye, missis, thank ye, we will that.' The two small faces looked up at her and smiled.

'I'll see you down the stairs, Mr Gibbons,' I said.

On the descent I tickled the furry cheek resting on the man's shoulder and heard for the last time the rich purring. On the front door step we shook hands and they set off down the street. As they rounded the corner of Trengate they stopped and waved, and I waved back at the man, the two children and the cat's head looking back at me over the shoulder.

It was my habit at that time in my life to mount the stairs two or three at a time but on this occasion I trailed upwards like an old man, slightly breathless, throat tight, eyes prickling.

I cursed myself for a sentimental fool but as I reached our door I found a flash of consolation. Helen had taken it remarkably well. She had nursed that cat and grown deeply attached to him, and I'd have thought an unforeseen calamity like this would have upset her terribly. But no, she had behaved calmly and rationally. You never knew with women, but I was thankful.

It was up to me to do as well. I adjusted my features into the semblance of a cheerful smile and marched into the room.

Helen had pulled a chair close to the table and was slumped face down against the wood. One arm cradled her head while the other was stretched in front of her as her body shook with an utterly abandoned weeping.

I had never seen her like this and I was appalled. I tried to say something comforting but nothing stemmed the flow of racking sobs.

Feeling helpless and inadequate I could only sit close to her and stroke the back of her head. Maybe I could have said something if I hadn't felt just about as bad myself.

You get over these things in time. After all, we told ourselves, it wasn't as though Oscar had died or got lost again – he had gone to a good family who would look after him. In fact he had really gone home.

And, of course, we still had our much-loved Sam, although he didn't help in the early stages by sniffing disconsolately where Oscar's bed used to lie, then collapsing on the rug with a long lugubrious sigh.

There was one other thing, too. I had a little notion forming in my mind, an idea which I would spring on Helen when the time was right. It was about a month after that shattering night and we were coming out of the cinema at Brawton at the end of our half-day. I looked at my watch.

'Only eight o'clock,' I said. 'How about going to see Oscar ?'

Helen looked at me in surprise. 'You mean – drive on to Wederly ?'

'Yes, it's only about five miles.'

A smile crept slowly across her face. 'That would be lovely. But do you think they would mind ?'

'The Gibbons ? No, I'm sure they wouldn't. Let's go.'

Wederly was a big village and the ploughman's cottage was at the far end a few yards beyond the Methodist chapel. I pushed open the garden gate and we walked down the path.

A busy-looking little woman answered my knock. She was drying her hands on a striped towel.

'Mrs Gibbons ?' I said.

'Aye, that's me.'

'I'm James Herriot – and this is my wife.'

Her eyes widened uncomprehendingly. Clearly the name meant nothing to her.

'We had your cat for a while,' I added.

Suddenly she grinned and waved her towel at us. 'Oh aye, ah remember now. Sep told me about you. Come in, come in!'

The big kitchen-living room was a tableau of life with six children and thirty shillings a week. Battered furniture, rows of much-mended washing on a pulley, black cooking range and a general air of chaos.

Sep got up from his place by the fire, put down his newspaper, took off a pair of steel-rimmed spectacles and shook hands.

He waved Helen to a sagging armchair. 'Well, it's right nice to see you. Ah've often spoke of ye to t'missis.'

His wife hung up her towel. 'Yes, and I'm glad to meet ye both. I'll get some tea in a minnit.'

She laughed and dragged a bucket of muddy water into a corner. 'I've been washin' football jerseys. Them lads just handed them to me tonight – as if I haven't enough to do.'

As she ran the water into the kettle I peeped surreptitiously around me and I noticed Helen doing the same. But we searched in vain. There was no sign of a cat. Surely he couldn't have run away again? With a growing feeling of dismay I realized that my little scheme could backfire devastatingly.

It wasn't until the tea had been made and poured that I dared to raise the subject.

'How—' I asked diffidently. 'How is – er – Tiger ?'

'Oh he's grand,' the little woman replied briskly. She glanced up at the clock on the mantelpiece. 'He should be back any time now, then you'll be able to see 'im.'

As she spoke, Sep raised a finger. 'Ah think ah can hear 'im now.'

He walked over and opened the door and our Oscar strode in with all his old grace and majesty. He took one look at Helen and leaped on to her lap. With a cry of delight she put down her cup and stroked the beautiful fur as the cat arched himself against her hand and the familiar purr echoed round the room.

'He knows me,' she murmured. 'He knows me.'

Sep nodded and smiled. 'He does that. You were good to 'im. He'll never forget ye, and we won't either, will we mother ?'

'No, we won't, Mrs Herriot,' his wife said as she applied butter to a slice of gingerbread. 'That was a kind thing ye did for us and I 'ope you'll come and see us all whenever you're near.'

'Well, thank you,' I said. 'We'd love to – we're often in Brawton.'

I went over and tickled Oscar's chin, then I turned again to Mrs Gibbons. 'By the way, it's after nine o'clock. Where has he been till now ?'

She poised her butter knife and looked into space.

'Let's see, now,' she said. 'It's Thursday, isn't it ? Ah yes, it's 'is night for the Yoga class.'

24

I knew it was the end of the chapter when I slammed the carriage door behind me and squeezed into a seat between a fat WAAF and a sleeping corporal.

I suppose I was an entirely typical discharged serviceman. They had taken away my blue uniform and fitted me with a 'demob suit', a ghastly garment of stiff brown serge with purple stripes which made me look like an old-time gangster, but they had allowed me to retain my RAF shirt and tie and the shiny boots which were like old friends.

My few belongings, including Black's *Veterinary Dictionary*, lay in the rack above in a small cardboard suitcase of a type very popular among the lower ranks of the services. They were all I possessed and I could have done with a coat because it was cold in the train and a long journey stretched between Eastchurch and Darrowby.

It took an age to chug and jolt as far as London then there was a lengthy wait before I boarded the train for the north. It was about midnight when we set off, and for seven hours I sat there in the freezing darkness, feet numb, teeth chattering.

The last lap was by bus and it was the same rattling little

vehicle which had carried me to my first job those years ago. The driver was the same, too, and the time between seemed to melt away as the fells began to rise again from the blue distance in the early light and I saw the familiar farmhouses, the walls creeping up the grassy slopes, the fringe of trees by the river's edge.

It was mid-morning when we rumbled into the market place and I read 'Darrowby Co-operative Society' above the shop on the far side. The sun was high, warming the tiles of the fretted line of roofs with their swelling green background of hills. I got out and the bus went on its way, leaving me standing by my case.

And it was just the same as before. The sweet air, the silence and the cobbled square deserted except for the old men sitting around the clock tower. One of them looked up at me.

'Now then, Mr Herriot,' he said quietly as though he had seen me only yesterday.

Before me Trengate curved away till it disappeared round the grocer's shop on the corner. Most of the quiet street with the church at its foot was beyond my view and it was a long time since I had been down there, but with my eyes closed I could see Skeldale House with the ivy climbing over the old brick walls to the little rooms under the eaves.

That was where I would have to make another start; where I would find out how much I had forgotten, whether I was fit to be an animal doctor again. But I wouldn't go along there yet, not just yet . . .

A lot had happened since that first day when I arrived in Darrowby in search of a job but it came to me suddenly that my circumstances hadn't changed much. All I had possessed then was an old case and the suit I stood in and it was about the same now. Except for one great and wonderful thing. I had Helen and Jimmy.

That made all the difference. I had no money, not even a house to call my own, but any roof which covered my wife and son was personal and special. Sam would be with them, too, waiting for me. They were outside the town and it was a fair walk from here, but I looked down at the blunt toes of my boots sticking from the purple striped trousers. The RAF hadn't only taught me to fly, they had taught me to march, and a few miles didn't bother me.

I took a fresh grip on my cardboard case, turned towards the exit from the square and set off, left-right, left-right, left-right, on the road for home.